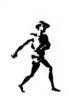

Personal Habit Control

Peter M. Miller, Ph.D.

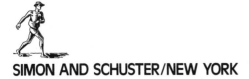

SIMON AND SCHUSTER/NEW YORK

Copyright © 1978 by Peter M. Miller
All rights reserved
including the right of reproduction
in whole or in part in any form
Published by Simon and Schuster
A Division of Gulf & Western Corporation
Simon & Schuster Building
Rockefeller Center
1230 Avenue of the Americas
New York, New York 10020
Designed by Libra Graphics, Inc.
Manufactured in the United States of America
1 2 3 4 5 6 7 8 9 10
Library of Congress Cataloging in Publication Data

Miller, Peter Michael, date.
Personal habit control.

1. Tobacco habit. 2. Obesity. 3. Alcohol abuse.
4. Habit. 5. Behavior modification. I. Title.
RC564.M54   616.8′6   78-10623

ISBN 0-671-24068-4

To GABRIELLE,
who created the idea for this book, inspired
me throughout its completion, and will always
be my healthiest and most treasured habit

Contents

ONE: You and Your Bad Habits   9

TWO: Why You Overindulge   21

THREE: Your Self-Control Strategy   43

FOUR: Breaking Your Bad Habits   77

FIVE: Personal Relaxation Training   107

SIX: You May Be Your Own Worst Enemy   137

SEVEN: Your Consummatory Style: Controlling
Your Eating, Smoking, and Drinking   159

EIGHT: How to Help Your Family and Friends
Help You   191

NINE: Getting Started   225

TEN: Permanent Personal Habit Control   239

CHAPTER ONE

——— You and Your Bad Habits

Personal Habit Control is an effective method of self-improvement that will enable you to gain permanent control over smoking, eating, and drinking. It is vastly different from other methods because of several simple factors. First, the self-help techniques of Personal Habit Control are straightforward and sensible. They aren't extreme or odd and they're easy to apply in your everyday life. Second, this approach is based on years of sound behavioral research on habit problems and not on some passing theory that is here today and will be gone tomorrow. Third, and perhaps most important of all, it works! And what's even more exciting, it can be the last habit-control program of your life!

In our fast-paced society in which time is so valuable and at times so scarce, we all look for the quickest and easiest solutions to our problems. This is especially true of habit patterns. For example, millions of dollars have been made by the developers of "miracle" diets, pills, and body wraps that offer "scientifically proven" ways to lose weight fast. Unfortunately, such methods are usually not based on objective scientific evidence, may or may not help an individual lose weight, and definitely will not result in permanent weight loss. In fact, over 80 percent of individuals who lose weight quickly using one of these methods will gain it back in three to four months. Many of these fads are also very detrimental to your over-all health. In addition, they give the user a false sense of hope, which is eventually followed by disappointment and despair when the procedure does not work as promised. In regard to the use of the so-called "diet pills" (usually amphetamines or amphetaminelike substances), the Council on Drugs of the American Medical Association has suggested that such medications are prescribed much too often by family physicians for weight control. In fact, the AMA concluded that these drugs are of limited usefulness in the treatment of obesity and can lead to drug dependence and certain undesirable effects on the cardiovascular system.

Similarly, numerous solutions to smoking and drinking habits have also been proposed, and again there is no evidence that any quick-and-easy solution to changing these patterns is effective in the long run.

Current research evidence suggests that the *only* way to gain total and permanent control over smoking, eating, and drinking is through major modifications in behavior patterns and life styles. This involves a process of unlearning old habits and learning new ones. Once you learn to objectively analyze your behavior patterns you can begin to implement a plan of change, using the specific self-help techniques described in subsequent chapters.

No one should enter on a program of behavior change lightly. You must be seriously committed to an intensive effort. For the first few weeks of your self-improvement program you will have to focus much of your attention on behavior changes. Typically, an individual begins such a program with a great deal of enthusiasm and concentrated effort. As the novelty wears off, motivation tends to decline. You may feel that you're not losing weight fast enough or that it's just not worth all the trouble to give up cigarettes or to control your drinking. You may feel that there are too many pressures from your job or your family to try to change your habits at this time. You may say that the cravings are just too strong for you to resist. In other words, you may be your own worst enemy for a while. Don't worry. Such thoughts and feelings and motivational problems are normal and are to be expected. While in the past these problems may have ruined your efforts at change, Personal Habit Control includes techniques of self-motivation to help you persist in the face of difficulties.

As your behavior-change efforts begin to pay off, your success will serve as its own reward to keep you going. You'll experience feelings of personal accomplishment that no pill or external "miracle cure" can give you. You'll realize that you have conquered your habit through your own persistent efforts. In addition, your health and personal appearance will improve. In other words, you'll not be just changing your eating, smoking, or drinking habits, you'll be embarking on a total reevaluation and change of your life style.

Basically, Personal Habit Control is derived from the belief that to understand and modify your habit patterns you don't have to delve into complicated causes of your behavior. Studies of how people learn habits indicate that behavioral patterns are governed primarily by the immediate circumstances surrounding their occurrence. Important elements of these circumstances include both the stimulus cues that trigger an episode of overeating, smoking, or excessive drinking and the immediate consequences of overindulgence.

Once you examine your behavior and pinpoint specific situational, social, emotional, cognitive, and physiological events associated with substance abuse, you will be ready to begin your program of habit change. Your plan of action will consist of three elements. First, you will develop alternative ways of responding to antecedent triggering events. For example, rather than smoke or overeat, you might use my Personal Relaxation Training technique (see Chapter 5) and learn to change the *style* of your habitual behavior pattern. With respect to alcohol, you would change not only how much you drink but also what you drink and how you drink (for example, the pace of your drinking). Finally, you will learn how to rearrange the consequences of your behavior so that they become more negative than positive.

Personal Habit Control is

1. Sensible
2. Easy to apply
3. Effective
4. Permanent!

You probably consider yourself to be a relatively normal, well-adjusted individual. You have your ups and downs, but basically you're in control of yourself. However, when it comes to "willpower," especially in regard to what you eat, smoke, and drink, you've been promising yourself to quit smoking, lose weight, or cut down on your drinking for years now. Somehow you make a valiant effort for a week or two, but then suddenly something happens. Perhaps it's a friend's birthday and you say to yourself, "One little piece of cake won't hurt me. I'll just have one small sliver!" Famous last words! Or perhaps you've just experienced an intense personal crisis in your life and you light a cigarette to obtain relief. Or perhaps you are too embarrassed to order a soda when everyone else is having a beer. Or maybe you say to yourself, "To hell with it! Why should I deprive myself when others can eat, drink, and smoke as much as they want? Anyway, I can start my new Personal Habit Control plan on Monday." Sound familiar? If it does, you're typical of millions of Americans. Many people have stopped smoking many times, have lost hundreds of pounds over their lifetimes, and have sworn repeatedly to drink less. Most people can adapt the now classic saying to each of their habit patterns: namely, "Quitting is easy. I've done it hundreds of times!!" As we all know, quitting *is* easy. But getting started again is even easier. *Permanent change is what's difficult, which is exactly why this book was written.*

Recent developments in the field of behavioral psychology can assist you in gaining permanent control over smoking, drinking, and eating habits. Fads aimed at quick-and-easy changes simply do not work. Permanent control can be developed only through over-all modifications in your basic habit patterns and general life style. Personal Habit Control will enable you to develop *effective* self-control and to learn behavioral, emotional, and cognitive alternatives to overeating, smoking, and excessive drinking. This process of behavior change involves learning to

1. Evaluate your habit patterns more systematically and objectively
2. Set goals for habit change
3. Develop a personal behavior-change plan
4. Control self-defeating thought patterns
5. Control external influences on habits (such as specific times in the day or situations that have been associated with heavy consumption)

6. Develop positive alternatives to old habit patterns
7. Deal with difficult interpersonal situations that make habit change more difficult (such as pressure from friends at a party to forget about your diet and enjoy the food)

This approach assumes that your habits are *learned* behavior patterns and that they can be *unlearned!* But before discussing the step-by-step method of *what* to do let's examine your habit patterns in more detail.

The Extent of Your Problem

You are certainly not alone in your concern over what you consume. About 40 million Americans are overweight and have tried again and again to lose weight. Approximately 30–40 percent of adult Americans smoke cigarettes. Approximately 10 percent of the 90 million consumers of alcohol in this country drink *too* much *too* often. Many people have all three habits. The latter group may find it the most difficult to change, since their habits are often related to one another. For example, remember the time you quit smoking and gained 20 pounds? How about the time you went on that water diet and started smoking three packs of cigarettes a day (not to mention all the time you spent running to the bathroom)?

Are These Habits Related?

Why, you may ask, is a book written about changing smoking, eating, *and* drinking habits? Someone who has three or four alcoholic drinks every evening isn't the same as someone who smokes three packs a day or someone who eats too many sweets. My answer is that they are very much alike, or at least their habits are. The basic premise of this book is that all of these habit patterns are developed and maintained in similar ways and that they can all be broken using similar self-control techniques.

In order to illustrate the relationship between these habits let me digress for a moment and briefly describe my own professional background as it relates to what I have termed the *addictive behaviors*. Several years ago I began studying and treating problem drinking. As I continued working with problem drinkers I quickly noticed that the techniques my colleagues and I were developing and studying were equally applicable to other habitual consummatory behaviors. This finally led to my establishing a Substance Abuse Clinic for problem drinkers, smokers, and overeaters. The clinic provided a unique opportunity to study the similarities between these behavior patterns in more detail. Unfortunately, most other behavioral researchers in the field were focusing on only one of these habits at a time. Although techniques being developed to help people control their drinking were also potentially helpful to smokers and dieters, professional communication in these fields was lacking. Thus a psychologist or physician specializing in weight control was not apt to keep up with the latest developments in the fields of smoking and alcohol abuse. On the other hand, new techniques of weight control were not readily accessible to clinicians in the smoking and alcohol fields.

To illustrate the commonality of *treatment* procedures for each of the addictive behaviors, I will briefly describe a technique that my colleague Dr. David Foy and I developed to help problem drinkers, which is directly applicable to smokers and overeaters as well. The procedure, known as *refusal training,* is a simple and practical technique designed to help problem drinkers resist the social pressure to have an alcoholic beverage. The procedure is an important one, since at least 25 percent of problem drinkers lose their "willpower" as a direct result of social pressure from friends to have a drink. Refusal training is designed to enable an individual either to refuse all drinks or, if he is merely trying to reduce his drinking, to refuse the second or third drink.

The technique can easily be adapted to the refusal of cigarettes and/or certain types of food. In fact, I am currently utilizing this exact procedure to help overweight patients handle offers of desserts and other high-calorie foods from well-meaning "friendly enemies." Once an individual learns this procedure he can apply it to a whole array of habit patterns that he is trying to control. The same is true for all of the behavior-change techniques throughout this book. They are easily learned and easily adapted to a variety of behavior patterns.

Health and Social Factors

It is frequently true that an individual will not admit to a problem habit or try to do anything about it until the habit results in a dire outcome. The heavy smoker may not feel strongly challenged to quit smoking until he has difficulty breathing or until his physician tells him that he has lung cancer. A problem drinker may not seek professional help until his wife leaves him or his boss threatens to fire him.

The detrimental effects on physical health of misusing food, cigarettes, and alcohol are well documented. Both obesity and smoking have been consistently linked to high blood pressure and heart disease. Studies sponsored by the National Heart and Lung Institute have found that people who smoke one pack of cigarettes a day are also less likely to survive a heart attack and are also more prone to emphysema and lung cancer. Obesity is associated with many health problems, including strokes, kidney ailments, diabetes, surgical complications, and breathing difficulties. The combination of smoking and being overweight is especally detrimental to your health. The overweight smoker triples his risk of a heart attack in comparison to the slim nonsmoker. In addition to causing cirrhosis of the liver, chronic excessive alcohol consumption, especially when combined with smoking, is often implicated in the development of cancer of the mouth, pharynx, larynx, and esophagus.

While the negative consequences of smoking are mainly health-related, obesity and alcoholism can have devastating social and psychological effects. Being overweight can drastically influence your social and family relationships and, most important, your feelings of self-worth and self-confidence. Heavy drinking can affect almost every aspect of your life. Job performance, mental abilities, driving performance, relationships with family and friends, sexual prowess, and memory suffer, either as immediate or as long-term results of consistent heavy drinking.

Overall, the knowledge that you are letting food, alcohol, or cigarettes control your life and happiness can cause a personal crisis. The belief that you have lost control often leads to apathy about the habit pattern, which in turn frequently puts an end to attempts at change.

How Much Is Too Much?

You may be asking yourself, "How much is too much? How do I know if I'm smoking, eating, or drinking too much?" Unfortunately, we can't always determine a problem habit on the basis of how much an individual consumes of a particular substance. Obviously, some people can have one alcoholic drink and get sick or act foolish, while others can have three or four with no ill effects. Some people can eat tremendous amounts of fattening foods and not gain weight, while others can eat a few cookies and almost see the pounds growing on them. In addition to the amount consumed we must also take into account the type of substance consumed and the frequency with which it is consumed. Thus an individual who smokes 30 low-tar and -nicotine filtered cigarettes has less of a problem habit than one who smokes 30 nonfiltered, high-tar and -nicotine cigarettes.

A second factor in defining "How much is too much?" relates to your reasons for substance use. For example, is your habit within your conscious control or do you "automatically" eat, smoke, and drink before you realize what you are doing? Do you eat, smoke, or drink to solve problems or ease tensions? Do you have frequent "cravings" when you try to do without your favorite substance? If so, you have a problem habit. These cravings often indicate a psychological addiction. That is, you are not *physically* addicted, but you find it very difficult to go without a cigarette, a drink, or your favorite food for any significant length of time. Physical addiction refers to the presence of physiological withdrawal symptoms when alcohol or cigarette consumption is stopped after a period of prolonged use. These symptoms can include irritability, tremulousness, anxiety, nausea, and sweating. In the case of alcohol, withdrawal symptoms may range from the hangover experienced by the social drinker to the DTs (delirium tremens) of the alcoholic, during which the addict hallucinates and trembles uncontrollably.

CHAPTER TWO

—— Why You Overindulge

Over the years numerous "experts" have proposed answers to why we consume substances that are known to be hazardous to our health. These explanations have served as the basis for professional advice on how best to control habit patterns. Unfortunately, human behavior is extremely complex, and no one explanatory system has been able to account for the development and maintenance of our habit patterns. Each simplistic explanation usually is expanded into an elaborate theory and is then swallowed hook, line, and sinker by millions of Americans. One amazing fact about human nature is that we seldom question the advice of anyone who claims to be an expert in his field. Once an individual writes his ideas into book form, his solutions to habit disorders are accepted as absolute fact. "After all," people say, "he must know what he's talking about—he wrote a book, didn't he?"

The ultimate proof of any theory lies in whether it can consistently explain certain behavior patterns and, more important, whether it can help to modify bad habit patterns. Proof must come not from a few individual testimonials from satisfied "customers" but from clinical research in which one method is compared with others to determine which is the 21 most effective. Effectiveness also must be judged by *permanent* behavior change and not merely by change over a two- or three-month period.

The major theories on which treatments have been based include the (1) physiological-heredity model, (2) sociological model, and (3) psychodynamic model. In this chapter I will present a newer, more practical, explanatory system known as the Personal Habit Control model. This model is based on the results of studies of habit-change techniques, and as such offers the reader a more valid system of personal habit control. First, let's briefly examine the three major theories of addictive behaviors upon which most past methods of change have been built.

Physiological-Heredity Model

A popular method of explaining habits is through a medical or disease model. Whereas a moralistic viewpoint places all of the blame on an individual for his bad habits, the disease model takes all of the personal responsibility for the habit away from him.

While medical explanations have been applied to all addictive habits, their application to alcohol problems has been by far the most elaborate. Up until very recently experts on alcohol abuse were concerned only with the older, chronic alcoholic. People were categorized into "social drinkers" and "alcoholics." Alcoholism is considered a *disease* by the medical profession and particularly by Alcoholics Anonymous.

Interestingly enough, alcoholism did not come to be labeled as a disease as the result of new research findings but rather as the result of the need for a change in the public's attitude. Historically, the general public has viewed alcoholism as a moral problem. With this view prevailing, alcoholics were seldom referred for professional help until several interested professional groups gave strong public support to the notion that alcoholism is a disease, and as such warrants medical treatment. Despite these claims, there is no solid evidence to support the idea that alcoholism is a physical disease caused by a physical abnormality. This is not to say, however, that alcohol abuse does not lead to some very serious medical problems. The point is that categorizing alcoholism as a disease does not adequately explain why some people drink too much. It may be, however, that hereditary and physiological factors increase an individual's susceptibility to the effects of alcohol. For example, because of low gastrointestinal tolerance you may find that any more than one or two drinks make you sick to your stomach. On the other hand, a friend of yours may find that he can drink excessively with no ill effects. His physiological tolerance for alcohol is not directly causing him to become a problem drinker, but given certain social and psychological circumstances, it may increase his chances of becoming an alcoholic.

Finally, when a physically addicted drinker tries to quit after a period of heavy drinking he may experience alcohol withdrawal symptoms—shaking, anxiety, nausea, sweating, headaches. His body is trying to adjust to the absence of alcohol, and although he can obtain temporary relief by taking another drink, he may eventually have to be hospitalized for medically supervised detoxification. A less severe form of alcohol withdrawal commonly experienced on Sunday morning is known as a hangover. You may find that another drink will make your head feel better temporarily. In this case, however, you are allowing your drinking to be induced by a physical event, that is, a decreased blood/alcohol level.

Generally speaking, hereditary and physiological influences only rarely cause an individual to be overweight. While obesity does tend to run in families, life-style patterns rather than heredity seem to be the culprit. If your parents ate the wrong kinds of food at the wrong times and in the wrong way, you would have learned these poor eating habits just by growing up in your family.

Differences in metabolism may account for the fact that some people seem to gain weight easily and others never gain no matter what they eat. In spite of this, however, overweight is ultimately caused by more food being consumed than is being burned up through activity. Regardless of your metabolism you still have to eat to gain weight. Your metabolism may put a limit on the amount you should eat to maintain a constant body weight, but it does not directly cause overweight. Along these lines, preliminary evidence suggests that if you have been overweight since childhood, you may have *more* fat cells than other people. Even when you lose weight you do not lose fat cells; they only get smaller. Therefore you may have a certain predisposition to gain weight. Again, however, this factor does not directly cause you to overeat.

There is certainly no innate physiological need or predisposition for people to smoke cigarettes. You can, however, train yourself to *need* cigarettes by becoming addicted to nicotine. Studies have shown that nicotine produces positive physiological effects on the body, among which is a dulling of the influence of unpleasant or stressful stimulation. And a smoker will actually alter the rate and duration of his smoking in relation to the nicotine content of his cigarettes. Consider the last time you switched to a low-tar and -nicotine cigarette in an attempt to cut down on your smoking. Behaviorally you probably responded to this change in nicotine content, perhaps without realizing it, by smoking faster and taking longer drags. You were compensating for the reduction in nicotine and attempting to maintain your old nicotine level. The same phenomenon occurs when a heavy drinker switches to weaker drinks. In the case of a very heavy smoker, smoking may be influenced by physical addiction. But physical addiction, although important, only partially explains why people smoke; nicotine substitutes in pill or gum form have not proven to be very effective. Psychological addiction, however, plays the most important role in smoking behavior.

Current evidence fails to demonstrate that habit patterns can be adequately explained on the basis of a disease model. While physiological predispositions, and particularly physical withdrawal factors related to addiction, must be taken into account in habit change, no magic pill or medical treatment will "cure" these addictive behaviors. Have you ever caught yourself saying:

"I can't do anything about my problem. I have a disease."

"Losing weight is impossible for me. I must have thyroid problems."

"When they find a cure for alcoholism I'll be able to quit drinking."

"It's not my fault that I smoke so much. I'm addicted to nicotine and my body needs cigarettes."

"Everybody in my family is overweight. My strong appetite is hereditary and there's nothing I can do about it."

If you have, you've succumbed to one of the major dangers inherent in disease explanations. You probably feel that you have lost control over your behavior, that something (a bio-chemical deficiency, perhaps?) is driving you to drink, smoke, or eat. The fact is that you have renounced personal responsibility for your habits. This type of thinking can be disastrous and can keep you from ever doing anything about your habit patterns. You must accept responsibility for change, because that's the only way you'll be successful.

Psychodynamic Model
Briefly, the psychodynamic model of addictive behaviors assumes that you consume substances to excess because of unconscious problems or unfulfilled needs. Psychoanalysts talk about oral dependency, tendencies toward self-destruction, the need to control others, fear of sex and repressed hostility. This model also assumes that certain personality types are more likely to abuse substances. The evidence for psychodynamic causes and specific personality profiles for those who eat, drink, and smoke too much is lacking. Even though psychological models are popular and are quoted frequently, there is little substantive evidence to support these explanations. Smokers, overeaters, and heavy drinkers represent a wide spectrum of personality types with a wide range of personal problems.

While intensive psychotherapeutic intervention may be helpful in selected cases, psychotherapy and psychoanalysis have not proven to be effective for most "addicted" persons. In the long run such a lengthy and costly individual approach to habit problems would not seem to offer an efficient or feasible solution to the problem.

Sociological Model
Another theory of substance abuse relates habit patterns to the social groups to which you belong. These include both small groupings, such as your family and close friends, and

larger ones, such as the society and culture in which you live. The attitudes, beliefs, and behavior of those around you have a great influence on whether or not you develop addictive habits and which ones you are more likely to develop. For example, the sociological model assumes that if, as you are growing up, your family, relatives and close friends all smoke heavily, you are likely to imitate this pattern. You will identify with these significant others in your life in an attempt to learn how to be an adult. Through a process known as *social role modeling* you will imitate many of their habits, both good and bad. You may learn poor nutritional habits in the same manner. Problem drinkers, for example, are most likely to come from families in which the parents are either alcoholics *or* teetotalers. This would seem at first glance to be a contradiction, but when you think about it, you'll realize that children of parents who drink in moderation are exposed to responsible drinking habits and, through social imitation, learn to drink in a similar manner. Children of alcoholic parents perceive continued examples of excessive use of alcohol as a way to solve problems or cope with life's tensions.

When both parents are completely abstinent, the child has no example of drinking, either good or bad. He must learn *how* to drink on his own, and the drinking patterns of his peer group take on greater importance. In this regard, the eating, drinking, and smoking patterns of your close friends can have an effect on your own habits. Whether you are aware of it or not, you will tend to smoke more if you socialize with friends who are heavy smokers, eat more with "gourmet" friends, and drink more with heavy-drinking friends. Give some thought to the groups of friends you have associated with over the years. You'll probably remember that you drank an awful lot more than you do now when you used to pal around with certain groups. What about your eating patterns when you were in that weekly dinner club or that bridge group?

Habit patterns are also determined by socioeconomic factors. Although addictive behaviors cut across all social strata, obesity and drinking problems are somewhat more prevalent among lower socioeconomic groups. Heavy drinking is more likely to occur in urban as opposed to rural families, and in broken homes. Cultural differences in life styles and attitudes can also serve as important determinants of habits. Jewish people have a low incidence of alcoholism, since the use of alcohol is circumscribed by their religious and cultural traditions, and heavy drinking is not tolerated by family and friends.

The United States generally has a history of ambivalent attitudes toward drinking. The drunk is often considered the life of the party! We joke and laugh about drinking and about who can drink someone else "under the table." On the other hand, we make halfhearted attempts to control intoxication, particularly on our highways. In the United States, drinking is not just encouraged, it is an integral part of our entire social system.

As a nation we also have more obese citizens than many other countries because of our abundance of food, our consumption of large quantities of sugar (more than 130 pounds per person each year), and our declining interest in physical activity. As a society becomes more "civilized," life becomes easier and obesity increases. Social eating customs also play a role in overeating. For example, more Italian Americans are obese than Americans of British ancestry. Pasta is simply more fattening than tea and crumpets!

The Banyankole of East Africa provide an extreme example of how attitudes toward overweight can influence behavior. Beginning at the age of eight, young girls are fed large quantities of milk, and at the same time their physical activity is severely restricted. They spend most of their time sitting, eating, and looking beautifully obese.

Thus social and cultural factors can set the stage for the development of certain habits. While it is not possible for you to drastically modify cultural influences on your habits, your awareness of more immediate social influences (for example, friends and family) can make a big difference in determining your eventual success in changing your overindulgence.

Personal Habit Control Model

The Personal Habit Control model is a nontheoretical system that developed its roots from behavioral psychology. It is based on the idea that habits are learned. Throughout your life you have learned how to talk, read, ride a bicycle, drive a car, *and* smoke, overeat, and drink alcohol. Within this frame of reference, habits can best be understood by examing the immediate circumstances surrounding their occurrence. More specifically, it is necessary to analyze the relationship among three events:

1. Antecedent cues
2. Habit pattern
3. Behavioral consequences

A particular set of antecedent cues occurs which triggers us to respond in a particular manner. Within the context of our discussion, we can either respond by consuming a substance or by engaging in a healthier, nonconsummatory behavior. One of the most important alternatives to overconsumption is complete muscular, cognitive, and physiological relaxation. This self-control method, which you will learn via my Personal Relaxation Training, is essential for permanent habit control.

In addition to its antecedents, our behavior produces an outcome, a change in us or in our immediate environment. Typically, the immediate consequence of your overconsumption is an extremely pleasurable one.

In the development of a habit pattern these three factors—antecedents, behavior, and consequences—become functionally related. That is, *behavior is determined by the relationship among these factors.* Let's assume that you feel bored, so you light up a cigarette or eat a plate of cheese and crackers. As a result, you momentarily feel satisfied and less bored. Without realizing it, you have begun to establish a pattern of relationships that will lead to an addictive habit pattern. The relationship involves a triggering event (boredom), the occurrence of a behavior (smoking/eating), and a positive outcome (temporary relief from boredom, a feeling of satisfaction or stimulation). From studies of behavior we know that the next time you feel bored the likelihood of smoking or eating increases because of these past associations. The more times these three factors occur together the more "automatic" your response becomes. In addition, whatever environmental cues are present during this sequence also become conditioned to your habit pattern. If your boredom ⟶ smoking ⟶ relief sequence frequently occurs while you are watching television, then television viewing becomes associated with smoking and can serve to support your habit. Then either boredom, television, or a combination of both can trigger your response of smoking a cigarette. Most of this self-conditioning occurs without our awareness.

The first step in controlling your habits is to identify the antecedent and consequent factors in your environment that are associated with them. We can categorize these factors as

1. Situational
2. Social
3. Emotional
4. Cognitive
5. Physiological

Situational Influences

Situational influences of behavior include specific visual, auditory, and time cues. Every time you eat, smoke, or drink, your behavior becomes associated with everything around you. As the result of this conditioning process, specific sights and sounds can elicit your particular consummatory behavior. Whereas previously the sequence of your eating was:

feelings of
hunger ⟶ snacking

it now becomes:

watching TV ⟶ feelings of hunger ⟶ snacking

Visual and auditory influences can be of two types. The first is direct sights and sounds of the substance you are trying to keep out of your mouth. For example let's suppose that you are sticking to your diet very well. You are not the least bit hungry and are not even thinking about eating. You open the refrigerator to put something away and you see the leftovers of the family's dessert staring you in the face. Just one piece of a chocolate layer cake. *Just one little piece!* The mere sight of that cake starts you thinking about food. Even though you argue with yourself, you can't get that cake out of your mind. You begin to feel "hungry." As you can see, the sight of food can be a powerful stimulus which may not necessarily drive you immediately to eating but may increase the chances that eventually you will eat. Overweight persons are much more susceptible to the influences of such "external" cues on their eating behavior than are individuals of normal weight. They are even much less accurate in judging when they are truly hungry in terms of physiological or "internal" cues than are other people. An interesting experiment was performed many years ago in which the stomach contractions of overweight and normal-weight subjects were measured. This was accomplished by having each individual swallow a balloon attached to a measuring device. The balloon was then inflated in the stomach so that stomach contractions would exert pressure on the balloon and be recorded. In this study, normal-weight individuals consistently reported feeling hungry only when stomach contractions were being recorded. However, overweight subjects reported hunger regardless of stomach contractions. They were less able to judge when stomach contractions were occurring. Subsequent studies have shown that the hunger of overweight persons can be "turned on," so to speak, simply by modifying external cues. That is, the obese will eat more if attractive food is available or if they feel that it is the right time to eat. Smokers and drinkers are probably overly responsive to the same "pull" from the environment. A newly abstinent ex-smoker may develop the craving to smoke after seeing numerous advertisements for cigarettes in a magazine. A formerly heavy drinker may experience the same urge after overhearing a conversation about how good a beer tasted to someone else.

Other external cues are not directly related to food, tobacco, and alcohol but have become influences because of a conditioning process. The relationship between coffee and cigarettes is a good example. Smoking while drinking coffee occurs so frequently with most people that these two become strongly associated. Once you give up smoking, coffee drinking (particularly in the morning or after a meal) will lead to the desire for a cigarette. Therefore one reason why a smoker smokes is the mere presence of certain conditioned external cues.

The time of day can also trigger a habit pattern. Examine the time periods of the day when you are more likely to practice your addiction. If you are a drinker, perhaps the hours between 5:30 and 7:00 P.M. are your drinking time. This would be particularly true if you are in the habit of coming home from work and having three or four drinks before dinner. When you try to quit or cut down, this time period will be your most difficult one. However, you can learn how to identify time influences and how to counteract them by changing your daily routine and by utilizing Personal Habit Control techniques.

Social Influences

"Oh, come on, have another helping of potatoes!" "All that research on smoking and health is a lot of baloney. Go ahead and light up. It hasn't killed me, has it?" "Hey, Jane, how about one for the road? You'll sleep better." Sound familiar? The role that other people play in your habits should never be underestimated. In fact, most failures in habit control occur as the direct result of well-meaning sabotage from others.

As you recall specific events that immediately preceded

your loss of habit control in the past you will discover that these events frequently involved other people. Occasionally you succumbed to temptation as the direct result of the encouragement or insistence of others. Your spouse may say, "You've done so well on your diet this week, give yourself a reward, a night off. We'll go to that great new Italian restaurant over on Fourth Street." In such cases the "friendly enemy" is often motivated by love and affection. This is particularly true with food. You may say to yourself, "How can I disappoint him? I don't want to hurt his feelings, so I'll go out and splurge just this once!" Unfortunately, once may be just enough to demolish your whole dietary program. The pound or two you gain at the restaurant may also be just discouraging enough to lessen your motivation to continue dieting.

You may have found that when others try to "help" you change your habits you quickly lose your motivation. The following example illustrates this phenomenon. Gary is a thirty-six-year-old junior executive who is energetic, ambitious, and determined to get ahead. His wife, Sharon, is very conscious of her role in helping Gary succeed. She is a very status-minded individual who makes it a point to lunch with the wives of other executives and give relaxed dinner parties for the "right" people in the company. Lately Sharon has become concerned over Gary's drinking and mentions it to him. Gary has noticed that over the last few years he has been drinking more and more. He usually has two to three drinks every evening before dinner and occasionally one or two more after dinner. Gary knows that during his business lunches with clients or colleagues he has been drinking too much. He worries that his drinking may begin to affect his dealings with clients. At the last two company parties Gary got so drunk that when he woke up the next morning he couldn't even remember what had happened. Gary decides to consciously limit his drinking, and he talks to Sharon about his plan. During the first few days of his Personal Habit Control program Gary does quite well. He limits his drinking to one cocktail before lunch and one before dinner—none before bedtime. On the fifth day of his program he arrives home from work and begins to fix his usual drink. Sharon says, "Gary, that drink looks a little strong. Don't you think you should pour out some of the Scotch and add more water? Here, let me do it for you." Gary notices that after this episode he feels like having a second drink. He finishes his first and fixes another. On Saturday, after mowing the lawn, Gary goes to the refrigerator for a beer. All of the beer is missing. Sharon comes in and informs him that in order to "help" him control his drinking she has given the beer to a neighbor. This results in Gary's fixing himself two strong Scotches and water. The conclusion of this example is that Sharon's attempts at helping him are a direct negative influence on his drinking. Gary's recognition of this functional A (antecedent) $\longrightarrow$ B (behavior) $\longrightarrow$ C (consequence) relationship is the first step in successful habit control.

In this case Sharon's reactions serve as antecedent events that trigger drinking *and* consequent events. The sequence is now likely to recur under similar circumstances. The positive or negative influence of a social consequence can be determined only by examining the precise relationship between the habitual behavior and a specific social outcome that that behavior produces. Let's suppose that every time Gary limits his drinking his wife says something like, "Oh, Gary, I'm so glad you are having only one drink tonight." Superficially, it would seem that this supportive comment should help Gary control his drinking, but we may find that when his wife responds in this manner he is more likely to have more than just one drink. In reality, her comments are not having a positive effect. This is important information in helping Gary and his wife develop a plan that will succeed. Other reactions of Sharon's that are more likely to result in increased habit control must be determined. This determination is based on Gary's own observation of relationships between his alcohol consumption and specific reactions that occur in response to his drinking. In subsequent chapters we will discuss how a person like Gary can use this information to develop a Personal Habit Control plan for himself.

Emotional Influences
Emotions can serve as strong influences over habit patterns. Emotions are particularly involved in sudden "binge" episodes during which the dieter gorges himself, consuming thousands of calories in a short period of time. Inability to cope effectively with stress can lead to the consumption of thousands of calories in one day. In the same way, the drinker consumes enough alcohol to obliterate all feeling, and the smoker smokes until his throat is sore. Emotional bingeing engenders feelings of guilt and self-condemnation, which in turn precipitate even more consumption.

In conducting a follow-up study of participants in a smoking clinic, Dr. Ovide Pomerleau, of the University of Pennsylvania, uncovered the importance of emotions in smoking. One year after the clinic ended he compared those who were completely abstinent with those who had resumed smoking. He found that those who had relapsed were much more likely to be "negative affect" smokers. This term refers to people who smoke in response to negative emotions, such as frustration, tension, boredom, depression, anger, impatience, and fatigue.

It could be that these smokers simply have developed a strong association between negative feelings and cigarette consumption. It may also be that these individuals have more problems in their lives to cause them more negative emotions than other people. In any event, learning to control emotions is a necessary precursor to habit control, particularly for "negative affect" smokers.

In a follow-up study of dieters, Dr. Gloria Leon and Dr. Karen Chamberlain, of Rutgers University, reported similar results. They found that 50 percent of dieters who had regained weight lost a year previously reported that they ate primarily in response to anger, boredom, loneliness, and tension. It is interesting to note, however, that this group also ate in response to excitement and extreme happiness. Thus they were both "*negative* affect" and "*positive* affect" eaters. The main triggering agent appeared to be emotional arousal, no matter what form it took. In contrast to this eating pattern, nonoverweight individuals typically eat because of hunger and enjoyment of food.

Anger is a specific emotion that is one of the major precipitants of loss of habit control. Anger can result in excessive substance use in an attempt to obtain emotional relief or to retaliate against the target of the anger. For example, certain occupations cause constant frustration and necessitate continued suppression of anger. Salespeople must be tactful with obnoxious customers, and junior executives must inhibit the impulse to tell the boss what they really think of him. Drinking becomes a means of letting go, of releasing pent-up emotions. Alcohol can neutralize anger by fostering an "I don't give a damn" attitude. In fact, heavy drinkers are often people who, because of their jobs or their personalities, are not able to express anger directly. In my own studies of alcohol abuse I have found that people who suppress anger are much more likely to abuse alcohol than those who let their feelings out.

Depression, boredom, and loneliness are other enemies of the habit controller. Having nothing to do or feeling lonely can lead to substance use in an effort to obtain emotional stimulation. The relationship between depression and habits is a rather complex one. For example, *moderate* drinkers usually experience temporary relief from depression or anxiety when they have one or two drinks. However, as the amount of alcohol consumed increases above seven or eight ounces, significant increases in depression and anxiety occur. After several years of very heavy drinking, alcohol begins to exert a different influence on the drinker. Unpleasant moods become *more* severe even after relatively low doses of alcohol. The alcoholic is fighting a losing battle by drinking to relieve depression and tension. He'll simply feel more depressed and more anxious with each successive drink. These negative feelings in turn precipitate even more drinking in a futile attempt to obtain emotional relief.

Depression and overeating also have a complex relationship. While *loss* of appetite is considered one of the classic symptoms of depression in most people, many overweight individuals react to depression in just the opposite way. They eat much more than usual and often become caught up in emotional-binge eating. While overeating produces some short-term relief, it eventually engenders guilt and more depression. The emotional eater becomes involved in the same frustrating cycle as the problem drinker.

Depression also functions in a more insidious way to undermine your habit-control efforts. This is especially true during the first few weeks of habit control, when you must be most vigilant. Recent studies indicate that depression interferes with self-control and restraint. It is often accompanied by feelings of powerlessness, of helplessness. You feel overpowered by the world, a pawn of your environment, with little internal control over yourself or anything around you. These are just the opposite kinds of feelings from those you must develop and maintain.

When depressed or upset, you must be more on your guard. You must determine what emotions occurring under what circumstances are most likely to interfere with your habit control. You *can* learn to control negative emotional arousal and the cravings associated with it. In Chapter 5, I will teach you a specific method of emotional control known as Personal Relaxation Training. Through this procedure, complete and total bodily relaxation, you will learn to control your emotions and your urges to overconsume.

Cognitive Influences

Thinking has often been referred to as nothing more than subvocal speech. Our thoughts are what we tell ourselves. We often tell ourselves some pretty peculiar things, especially about our habits. If you can accept the notion that thinking is self-talk, then you can begin to listen to what you are saying to yourself. The results may be startling. You will probably find that on numerous occasions you have actually talked yourself into having a drink, cigarette, or food. You will also find that you provide yourself with acceptable excuses, rationalizations, for engaging in your bad habit. How many of the following thoughts sound familiar to you?

> "Why should I have to diet? Jane is as skinny as a rail and can eat anything she wants. It's just not fair. I'm not very overweight anyway."

> "I've been smoking for twenty years and I'm in good health. Anyway, it wouldn't do any good if I stopped now. The damage is already done."
> "I just don't have the willpower to quit."
> "I'll quit in January. With all of the holidays coming up, it would be impossible to cut down on my drinking."
> "I have too many problems to quit. I'm tense and depressed all of the time. It wouldn't be good for me to quit."
> "I'll faint if I don't have a few cookies. My system can't take the few calories on this diet."
> "I've got something physically wrong with me. My system must need alcohol or I wouldn't drink so much."
> "If it weren't for my job I'd quit tomorrow. I have to drink with my customers or I'd lose some of my accounts."

These thoughts can lead directly to substance use. While we all say these things to ourselves from time to time, you *can* learn to recognize and control these thought patterns more effectively.

Finally, guilty thoughts over a brief relapse can be a very negative influence. A smoker who has one cigarette will think, "Well, I've blown it now. I've ruined everything I've accomplished for the past month. I'll just buy a pack and try to quit again next week." *One* cigarette has led to a feeling of guilt over "failure," which in turn has led to more smoking. This irrational thinking is characteristic of most of us. We think in terms of absolutes. We say that we are either "off" or "on" a diet, smoking or not smoking. This is nonsense! This is the kind of thinking that serves as an excuse to continue old habits. One cigarette does not mean failure. The ex-smoker can stop after one cigarette or after one puff of that cigarette, for that matter. You must give yourself credit for those times when you resisted cigarettes.

Physiological Influences

Physiological influences refer to any physical discomfort that consistently occurs prior to excessive substance use. These include headaches, backaches, fatigue, dizziness, tremulousness, and other such symptoms. Often substance use is an attempt to obtain relief—drinking alcohol to relieve pain, eating to relieve fatigue, smoking to relieve tension caused by abstention from smoking. In the latter case the precipitant event is actually one of the physiological symptoms of cigarette withdrawal.

CHAPTER THREE

Your Self-Control Strategy

Now that you are aware of the possible influences on your addictive behavior, let's get a little more personal. Generalities are fine to get a point across, but to modify your behavior successfully you must focus on specifics.

When I first meet with people who are beginning to change their habits I usually ask a very simple question: "*Why* do you smoke?" Their answers are invariably the same. It's usually something vague, such as "I just get this urge to smoke" or "It's nerves—I just get all tense inside." Yes, perhaps these are partial causes for the habit pattern. However, the basis for a habit is never that simple. If it were, there would be no need for this book.

People simply do not know what specifically triggers and maintains their habit patterns. You must begin to develop a personal behavioral analysis of your habit based on self-observation. Basically, you must learn to identify important determinants of your behavior and predict their occurrence. In this way you can plan a strategy of self-control and have it ready when needed.

Self-Observation

The simplest way to identify what influences your habits is to observe your own behavior. You must, however, be sys-   43 tematic in your observations. Self-observation will involve writing down certain details of your behavior. Now, don't panic. You may say, "I'm not the kind of person who is compulsive enough to write down all kinds of stuff about my eating. I've never been very orderly or organized." If you want to make changes in your habit you must make an initial commitment to undergo some discomfort and do things differently. This is extremely important. Just say to yourself, "I know it will be difficult, but I can and will do it." *Never* say, "I'll *try*." "Try" is a word that you should eradicate from your vocabulary. Every time you catch yourself saying it, use the word "will" instead. Now say, "*I will do it.*"

Don't say:	*Do* say:
I'll try.	I will!
If I succeed . . .	*When* I succeed . . .
I'll give it my best.	I will do it!
I hope I can do it.	I'm positive I can do it!

Content

To begin your behavioral self-analysis you will need index cards or several sheets of paper. Set up each card or piece of paper with columns marked with the following headings: date, time, place, activity, people, and feelings or thoughts. Your cards should resemble the one shown in Figure 1. If you are observing your drinking or eating patterns, you might need only one index card per day. Because smoking involves so many separate episodes each day, you may decide to use longer sheets of paper or more index cards per day.

At this stage of your personal behavioral analysis do not try to interpret your behavior or try to figure anything out. Just be an observer. But be an accurate one.

Figure 1 SAMPLE SELF-OBSERVATION CARD

Date	Time	Place	Activity	People	Feelings or Thoughts

Every time you engage in your habit write down: (1) the time, (2) your specific location, such as the kitchen, back yard, bathroom, or living room, (3) what you are specifically doing (if you are talking to a friend and drinking coffee at the same time, write down both activities), (4) who is with you, and (5) what thoughts or feelings you had immediately prior to your behavior. At times you may feel simply neutral, with no particular thoughts or feelings. In that case just leave the space blank.

With alcohol or food you should add a column specifying the *type* and *amount* of substance consumed. In addition, when monitoring food intake, rate your degree of hunger prior to eating on a 5-point scale. A rating of 0 would indicate no hunger, and 5 would indicate extreme hunger. You may be amazed to learn that much of your eating occurs after ratings of 0 and 1. A sample eating diary would look like Figure 2.

Procedure

The best procedure for self-observation is to record each instance of consumption as it occurs or immediately after it occurs. Therefore, keep your record sheet with you at all times. You may think: "Well, that's going to look cute! I'll be eating in a restaurant with friends and I'll say, 'Excuse me, I'm keeping a diary of my eating experiences. You know— what I do when I'm eating, whom I'm with, that sort of thing. Interesting, isn't it?' " Rather than risk being labeled as "a bit strange" you can write down the pertinent information later when you're alone. However, *be very careful;* it is very easy to forget little details about your eating episode that can be very important.

With eating and drinking, you should record your behavior consistently for at least a week or two to obtain an accurate picture. Since smoking is so much more time-consuming to observe in this way, you might choose to monitor your smoking every other day rather than daily. For our purposes here it is important that you observe a full day of behavior rather than selected episodes during the day or only during the morning or evening.

You may notice that merely by observing and recording your behavior you are modifying it. The process of analyzing your habit pattern is making you more aware of the situations in which you smoke, eat, or drink, and this awareness gives you an advantage. The first step in controlling your behavior is to identify the situations in which it occurs. Since your habit is so strong, many episodes of consumption occur automatically, without your awareness. It's like the patellar tendon reflex, or knee jerk. When the doctor hits your knee with his hammer, your leg goes up. Awareness is a basic necessity for habit change. You must be aware not only of the fact that you are puffing on a cigarette but also of the sequence of events leading up to that event. The sequence of events might be: seeing someone else light a cigarette, taking a cigarette from your pack, putting the cigarette in your mouth, taking out your lighter, lighting the cigarette, taking a puff. The earlier in this chain of events that you are aware of what is happening, the more control you will have.

Some years ago I tried an interesting experiment with a group of college students who wanted to stop the habit of biting their nails. The treatment was simply one of making them more aware of each step in the sequence of their behavior. I first asked them to count the number of times they actually bit their nails each day for one week. During the

Figure 2 SAMPLE EATING DIARY
Friday, June 3, 1977

Time	Food	Calories	Hunger Rating	Location	Activity	People	Thoughts and Feelings
8:00 A.M.	8 oz. orange juice	110	2	Kitchen	Reading newspaper	Husband	Depression
	3 strips bacon	72					
	2 eggs	140					
	2 English muffins	300					
	2 cups coffee	0					
10:30	2 doughnuts	225	4	Living room	Ironing	Alone	"I hate ironing. I'd rather be playing tennis."
	2 cups coffee	0					
12:30 P.M.	Broiled chicken	154	2	Restaurant	Talking to friend	Friend	Relaxed
	Small potato	65					
	Salad	80					
	½ cup beans	18					
	Iced tea (no sugar)	0					

Figure 2 SAMPLE EATING DIARY (Cont.)
Friday, June 3, 1977

Time	Food	Calories	Hunger Rating	Location	Activity	People	Thoughts and Feelings
4:30	Ice cream cone (double dip)	450	0	Car	Driving	Alone	"Maybe if I eat this now, I won't eat as much for supper."
5:30	5 pieces cheese 5 crackers	400 55	1	Kitchen	Preparing meal	Alone	
6:00	Small steak Salad ½ cup peas Gelatin	550 75 58 81	3	Dining room	Talking to family	Family	Relaxed
9:30	1 cup peanuts 1 soft drink	1200	1	Family room	Watching TV	Husband	Bored

second week they recorded the number of times they put their fingers in their mouths. During subsequent weeks I had them monitor the number of times they raised their hands to their mouths, raised their hands above their waists, or thought about raising their hands to bite their nails. The results indicated that as the students became more aware of each component of the nail-biting sequence they developed excellent control. In fact, control increased as awareness developed regarding progressively earlier elements of the behavioral sequence. Students monitoring either urges or hand-raisings bit their fingernails much less often than those monitoring nail-biting *per se*.

The use of self-observation and behavioral awareness as self-control techniques will be described in Chapter 4.

How to Interpret Your Behavioral Self-Analysis

Now that you have all this wonderful information about yourself, how can it help you? You must first examine your records carefully for trends and associations among categories. As we examine each major category, prepare a summary sheet detailing the results of your self-analysis.

DATE

By recording dates you can determine if you are more likely to engage in your habit on different days of the week. Perhaps you smoke less on Saturday and Sunday, when you are more physically active. Perhaps you eat and drink *more* on weekends. Maybe you find that you eat more on Monday and Tuesday. Look over your records carefully and jot down on your summary sheet (1) the days when you are most likely to smoke, eat, or drink and (2) the days when you are least likely to overindulge.

TIMES OF THE DAY

Now let's examine each day in more detail. Divide the day into six time intervals:

> Awakening to 10:00 A.M.
> 10:00 A.M. to 1:00 P.M.
> 1:00 P.M. to 4:00 P.M.
> 4:00 P.M. to 7:00 P.M.
> 7:00 P.M. to 10:00 P.M.
> 10:00 P.M. to retiring

Count the number of cigarettes smoked, amount of food consumed, or alcoholic beverages drunk in each time interval. On your summary sheet write the two time intervals associated with your greatest consumption and the two associated with your least consumption. If you are a heavy consumer you will probably find that you begin smoking, drinking, or eating very early in the day and continue until very late in the evening. Overeating usually occurs at very specific time intervals; overweight people usually overindulge in the late afternoon or late evening. If you are a binge eater you will probably find that you overeat very late at night, perhaps from 10:00 P.M. to 2:00 A.M. In fact, a binge eater, much like a binge drinker, can consume moderate amounts of food during the day, even eating less than most people during regular meals. During an emotional crisis, however, binge eaters have been known to consume as many as 20,000 calories in one day! That's more than most people would eat in a whole week's time.

PLACES

Where do you do most of your smoking, eating, or drinking? Do you eat mostly at home or out at parties and restaurants? If it's at home, do you eat in the kitchen, living room, bedroom, or den? While you may eat most of your meals at the kitchen or dining room table, you may snack or even eat some meals in the family room while watching television. Or perhaps on the back porch while reading. Actually, part of your habit problem is that you eat, smoke and drink in a wide variety of places. Each place, then, becomes associated with your addictive behavior and can serve as a stimulus for overindulgence. Write down at least five places in which you overindulge and five others in which you seldom or never indulge in your habit.

ACTIVITIES

Look over all the activities associated with your consumption. The following is a list of activities that are frequently associated with overeating, smoking, and drinking. Indicate how often you engage in your habit along with these activities.

	Never or Seldom	Occasionally	Frequently
While driving			
After physical activity			
After waking			
Before retiring			
With coffee			
With alcohol			
While preparing a meal			
During a meal			
After a meal			
Watching TV			
Talking on phone			
While reading			

	Never or Seldom	*Occasionally*	*Frequently*
During housework			
Writing letters			
Reading mail			
Taking a bath			
Taking a walk			
Listening to music			
After sexual activity			
At my desk			
During work break			
In conferences or meetings			
During a party			
With others who smoke			
In a bar			
Sewing, knitting, etc.			
Other activities:			

After rating your behavior pattern, list on your summary sheet all activities checked in the *Frequently* column and all activities checked in the *Never or Seldom* column.

PEOPLE

Do you eat, smoke, or drink alone or with other people? Calculate the approximate percentage of occasions during which you consume your favorite substance by yourself and with others. Write this information on the summary sheet. Now let's examine the types of people associated with your habit. Write down the categories of people (spouse, close

friend, coworker, acquaintance, customer, daughter, others)
who were present on more than one occasion of your in-
dulgence. Write specific names if they are people who are
close to you or whom you see frequently. Next to each name
indicate whether the person also has your habit. Then write
next to each name whether or not that person is one of your
"friendly enemies." For example, people qualify as friendly
enemies for dieters by (1) urging you to eat, (2) eating
high-calorie foods in your presence, (3) consistently saying
or doing things that anger or upset you. Thus your summary
list may look like this:

> *People*
> Husband, George—friendly enemy: eats very little
> Sister, Sarah—friendly enemy: loves to eat

FEELINGS OR THOUGHTS

It is important to determine if specific feelings or thoughts
trigger substance abuse. Again, examine your records. Do
you see any pattern? For example, how often were you feeling
tense or bored or depressed prior to having a drink or lighting
a cigarette. Food, cigarettes, and alcohol can all function
to relieve these feelings *temporarily*. On the other hand, many
people drink or eat more when they are perfectly content and
happy. Ironically, many heavy drinkers consume the most
alcohol when everything in their lives is going extremely well.

What thoughts were associated with consumption? Look
over your cards and try to organize these thoughts into categories. Are they self-put-downs, such as "I'll never be able to
complete this assignment. I just don't have what it takes."
Perhaps they're rationalizations, such as "Just one drink will
give me the confidence I need to tell Jack what I really think
of him."

Interrelationships Among Factors

Now that you have analyzed each factor separately, let's look at relationships among factors. Seldom, if ever, is your behavior determined by one specific situation, thought, or feeling. Rather, overconsumption is the result of the influence of combinations of factors occuring within a relatively brief period of time. Identification of the combination of events that is most likely to lead to smoking, drinking, or eating is absolutely mandatory for successful habit control. When a person simply goes on a diet to lose weight he or she never becomes aware of these influences. When a person goes off the diet, weight is usually regained because the factors that influenced overeating prior to the diet are still in operation.

Once combinations of events associated with habits are identified, you can begin to predict when smoking, eating, or drinking is likely to occur. This is *extremely* important. Because if you know ahead of time that you are probably going to eat or smoke, you can take steps to control your behavior. In addition, once you have identified combinations of influences on your behavior, you can learn to change your life so that you either remove some of these influences from your surroundings or decrease their effects on you.

You must be able to make *probability statements* about your behavior. A probability statement is simply an educated guess regarding the chances of your drinking or not drinking, eating or not eating, smoking or not smoking, based on your past behavior under specific circumstances. Simply stated, past behavior in a particular situation is the best predictor of present and future behavior in that same situation. Because human behavior is so complex we can never predict its occurrence with 100 percent accuracy. But it is amazing how consistently some behavior can be predicted on the basis of probabilities. This may shock you, and you may resist the idea that your behavior—the behavior of a rational, intelligent human being—can be so predictable. Well, it's true, and because it's true, your efforts at behavior change will be a lot easier. If there were no logic to your habit patterns—that is, no predictability—there would be no way for you to ever modify your behavior. Habit patterns are extremely logical, and they can be studied as scientifically as the principles of physics or chemistry. In fact, I am going to teach you how to become your own personal behavioral scientist.

Next, let's look at the interrelationships in your self-observations and begin to develop probability statements. First, identify your High-Probability Antecedent Clusters— Hi-Pacs. A Hi-Pac consists of environmental, social, emotional, and cognitive factors that frequently occur together prior to excessive smoking, eating, or drinking. You may notice that you are very likely to eat on weekends during the evening hours, when you are alone and bored. Your High-Probability Antecedent Cluster, then, consists of two environmental factors (day and time), a social factor (being alone), and an emotional factor (boredom). When these events occur in combination your chances of overeating high-calorie foods are greatly increased. Perhaps if even one factor were modified, the probability of your eating would be decreased significantly. Perhaps during the morning hours on weekends when you are alone and bored you usually do *not* overeat. Or perhaps in the evening on a weekend when you are with someone else you are not likely to eat. If heavy drinking is your problem you may find that one of your Hi-Pacs includes the following components:

1. Argument with boss
2. Driving home from work with friends who want to stop off for a drink
3. Having no plans for the evening

Remember, the more specifically you can pinpoint exact combinations of events associated with heavy consumption, the easier it will be to control your habit. Certainly you will have more than one Hi-Pac. You will probably be able to identify several. Once you identify several such clusters, write them down on your summary sheet.

It is equally important to identify Low-Probability Antecedent Clusters (Lo-Pacs). A Lo-Pac is a combination of events associated with light consumption or with total abstinence. An example for an overeater would be:

1. Eating lunch with another dieter
2. Eating in a restaurant with several low-calorie selections on the menu
3. Having been complimented recently on my appearance

An example for an excessive drinker would be:

1. Driving home from work alone and avoiding passing a favorite bar
2. Having no money or credit cards in my possession
3. Having planned to take my son to a ball game upon arriving home

The Case of Dorothy

In order to illustrate this behavioral self-analysis procedure in more detail, let's examine the case of Dorothy, a smoker who is trying to quit. Dorothy is a forty-nine-year-old woman who is married, has two children in college, and works as an advertising executive in Chicago. She has been trying to quit smoking for months. Lately she has developed high blood pressure and emphysema and has been advised by her physician that she *must* stop smoking. Dorothy is upset and concerned over her health and has made a serious commitment to modify her smoking habit. She embarks on a self-observational study and keeps detailed records of her smoking pattern for two weeks. A sample day of her self-monitoring is presented in Figure 3. Her smoking on other days of the week is similar to this sample, with the exception of weekends. Dorothy finds that on weekends her smoking is reduced by about half. Overall, Dorothy's summary self-evaluation sheet looks like this:

Days
Monday through Thursday—most smoking
Friday through Sunday—least smoking

Times
7:30 A.M. to 10:00 A.M.—most smoking
12:00 M. to 4:00 P.M.—most smoking
10:00 A.M. to 12:00 M.—least smoking
7:00 P.M. to 12:00 P.M.—least smoking

Places
Car—most smoking
Office—most smoking
Restaurant—most smoking
Social gathering—most smoking
Bedroom—least smoking
Outdoors—least smoking
Dining room—least smoking

Activities
Driving—most smoking
Drinking coffee—most smoking

Drinking alcohol—most smoking
Business meetings—most smoking
Reading—least smoking
Walking—least smoking
Recreational activities—least smoking
Interacting with family—least smoking

People
Alone—40 percent
With others—60 percent
Coworkers: most are smokers
Customers: some smokers, some nonsmokers
Husband, George: nonsmoker, occasional friendly enemy
Friend, Martha: heavy smoker, friendly enemy

Feelings
Tension—most smoking
Boredom—most smoking
Relaxation—least smoking

Thoughts
Expectations that others will disapprove of me or the quality
of my work—most smoking
Negative motivational thoughts—most smoking: "What's the
use of quitting? Something's going to kill me eventually. I
might as well enjoy life from day to day."
Feelings of personal accomplishment—least smoking
Feelings of affection for my husband and children—least
smoking
Thoughts regarding the negative health consequences of con-
tinual smoking (shorter life and especially poorer quality of
life due to ill health)—least smoking

Interrelationships

High-Probability Antecedent Clusters

Cluster #1
1. Driving
2. Alone in car
3. Feeling tense
4. Thinking about work

Figure 3 DOROTHY'S BEHAVIORAL ANALYSIS OF HER CIGARETTE SMOKING

Time	Place	Activity	People	Feelings or Thoughts
7:30 A.M.	Bedroom	Getting out of bed	Husband	Sleepy
8:00	Kitchen	Breakfast coffee	Husband	——
8:20	Kitchen	Cleaning breakfast dishes	Husband	——
9:15	Car	Driving to work	Alone	Tense: "I have to present that big report today."
9:30	Car	Driving to work	Alone	"I hope the boss likes my presentation."
9:45	Office	Preparing for meeting	Alone	"I'll probably screw up in front of everybody."
10:10	Boardroom	Preparing for presentation	Business associates	"I should be better prepared."
10:30	Office	Drinking coffee, dictating	Alone	Tense
12:00	Restaurant	Drinking martini, discussing business	Business associate	Relaxed
12:40 P.M.	Restaurant	Drinking coffee after lunch	Business associate	——
12:55	Car	Driving back to work	Alone	——
1:45	Office	Drinking coffee	Business associate	——

Figure 3 DOROTHY'S BEHAVIORAL ANALYSIS (Cont.)

Time	Place	Activity	People	Feelings or Thoughts
3:45	Office	Drinking coffee	Alone	"I'll never be able to give up smoking."
4:30	Boss's office	Discussing account	Boss	"I bet he thinks I'm messing up this account."
5:00	Car	Driving home	Alone	
5:45	Car	Driving home	Alone	"I'd never be able to relax without cigarettes."
6:00	Living room	Drinking martini	Husband	————
6:20	Living room	Drinking martini	Husband	————
7:30	Dining room	Drinking after-dinner coffee	Husband	Relaxed
8:30	Family room	Watching TV	Alone	Bored
11:30	Porch	Drinking wine	Husband	Relaxed
12:30 A.M.	Bedroom	In bed, after sex	Husband	Relaxed

Cluster #2
1. Tuesday evening
2. Social gathering
3. Many smokers present
4. Having had two drinks

Cluster #3
1. Office
2. Between 8:00 and 10:00 A.M.
3. Drinking coffee
4. Feeling that boss has disapproved of me

Cluster #4
1. Visiting with Martha (best friend)
2. Urging by Martha to have just one cigarette
3. Thinking "One won't hurt me."

Low-Probability Antecedent Clusters

Cluster #1
1. Weekend
2. With family
3. No cigarettes in house
4. Positive comments from family about not smoking

Cluster #2
1. Sunday
2. Playing tennis or walking
3. Thinking about positive benefits of not smoking (e.g., breathing is easier)

Cluster #3
1. Weekday
2. Evening
3. Reading enjoyable book
4. Feeling relaxed

Cluster #4
1. Weekday
2. Evening
3. Social gathering with few smokers
4. Having told group that I have quit smoking

Setting Behavioral Goals—Analysis of Dorothy's Profile

Dorothy now has a much better picture of the kind of events that influence her smoking in both negative and positive ways. In order to utilize this information for her benefit Dorothy must set goals based on her behavioral analysis. These behavioral goals must be stated specifically and will be the targets of change.

First of all, let's examine some goals Dorothy might consider in each general category of influential events. Then we'll consider clusters in her Hi-Pacs and Lo-Pacs and set specific goals for these situations. The procedures necessary to accomplish these goals will be described in detail in subsequent chapters.

ENVIRONMENTAL GOALS

Environmental goals relate to the days, times, and places that influence smoking. Dorothy is most likely to smoke on weekdays between 7:30 and 10:00 A.M. and between 12:00 noon and 4:00 P.M.—at her office, in her car, at a restaurant, or at a social gathering. Therefore, at these times she must be on guard; she must plan strategies to change these patterns. Other environmental factors may play a part, such as the mere availability of cigarettes. Dorothy may consider the following environmental goals:

1. Reduce exposure to cigarettes, ashtrays, people who are heavy smokers, and cigarette advertisements.
2. Reduce coffee consumption—begin to substitute iced tea.

3. Change schedule in morning to reduce desire for cigarette—get up early and walk briskly for 30 minutes before breakfast.
4. Place "no smoking" signs around office; also remove ashtrays from office, or at least remove them from sight until a smoker visiting the office needs one.
5. Remove ashtray from car and put "no smoking" sign on dashboard.
6. Reduce alcohol consumption for at least 3 months or until smoking is under control.

SOCIAL GOALS

Dorothy is slightly more likely to smoke with others than when alone. She is also more likely to smoke (1) when in the presence of another smoker, (2) when another smoker encourages her to smoke, and (3) when someone, her husband perhaps, makes discouraging remarks. For example, he might say, "There you go, smoking again. I knew you had no willpower." This statement usually irritates Dorothy and leads her to smoke one or two additional cigarettes she might otherwise have done without. Dorothy's social goals might include

1. Telling all relatives, close friends, and coworkers that she has quit smoking forever and asking them never to offer her a cigarette
2. Learning how to refuse cigarettes gracefully, especially with her friend Martha
3. Learning to be more assertive in responding to negative comments from husband and others regarding her attempts at smoking control

EMOTIONAL AND COGNITIVE GOALS

Dorothy is most likely to smoke when tense or bored and least likely to smoke when relaxed. Therefore her goals might include

1. Learning the self-relaxation method
2. Analyzing specific situations that make her tense and trying to deal with them more effectively
3. Increasing the variety of nonconsummatory spare-time activities that provide satisfaction, enjoyment, and challenge

Dorothy is very susceptible to certain types of thoughts that lead to smoking. These thoughts consist of (1) negative self-evaluations, (2) expectations that others will not approve of or be pleased by the quality of her performance at work, and (3) positive benefits of immediate pleasure from smoking. On the other hand, she is least likely to smoke when thinking of her personal accomplishments, her family, and her health. Her cognitive goals might involve

1. Increasing thoughts about the health consequences of continued smoking and the health benefits of not smoking
2. Reconsidering her negative self-evaluations and her expectations of disapproval and retraining her thought patterns
3. Learning to recognize her negative motivational thoughts and rationalizations for what they are and replacing them with more positive thoughts (For example, replacing "I'm just too tense to live without cigarettes" with "I'm no more tense than most people. I can learn to relax without

cigarettes. It's just a matter of changing my life a bit").

From a positive standpoint, Dorothy can arrange for herself to be exposed to as many of her Low-Probability Antecedent Clusters as possible. This is especially true during the first two weeks of her Personal Habit Control plan, when the urge to smoke may be strongest.

Now let's take a specific Hi-Pac in Dorothy's life and establish goals for her for that one set of circumstances. What about Cluster #2? Of the four factors listed, Dorothy should determine which ones would be the easiest to modify. First of all, let's list all possible changes she could make, whether the goals we set are practical or not:

1. Refuse all social invitations.
2. Refuse all social invitations during the week.
3. During the first three weeks of new program, refuse all social invitations.
4. Avoid social gatherings with many smokers present.
5. While at social gathering avoid conversations with groups of people who are smoking.
6. Avoid all alcoholic beverages.
7. Limit drinking to one alcoholic beverage.
8. At the social gathering announce to as many people as possible, "I have given up smoking."

Of the goals listed, Dorothy must now decide which she is likely to accomplish and which are impractical. She might decide that she is not willing to give up social invitations. She might be willing, however, to avoid alcohol at parties, since she knows drinking will influence the probability of her smoking. If she wants a helpful clue, Dorothy might look for a Lo-Pac that involves a similar social situation and examine its components. Indeed, her Lo-Pac #4 indicates that if she is around only a few smokers and if she tells people at the party she has quit smoking, she is not very likely to smoke that evening. So Dorothy sets the following goals for herself, which she feels are realistic for her:

1. Try to converse mostly with other nonsmokers at the party.
2. Tell as many people as possible that I have quit smoking (in order to increase social pressure against smoking).
3. Avoid all alcoholic beverages—substitute soft drinks.

If this strategy fails, rather than give up, Dorothy would simply reevaluate her goals and establish new ones. She may have to become more drastic. She may decide to avoid all social events and refrain from all alcoholic beverages for two weeks and then gradually reexpose herself to these circumstances. The beginning of her smoking-control program, when urges are strong, may require more severe behavioral restrictions.

What about Hi-Pac #4? Again, let's consider solutions. Before reading the rest of this paragraph refer back to Dorothy's Hi-Pac #4 and give some thought to what behavior-change goals you might set for yourself if you were faced with the same set of circumstances. Now you know what you'd do; what has Dorothy decided to do? First of all, Dorothy does not want to give up her friendship with Martha. Martha, however, is a very persuasive individual who is also a heavy smoker. She enjoys getting together with Dorothy for coffee and cigarettes. Martha does not allow her children to see her smoking (apparently so they don't pick up the habit through imitation), and she therefore takes the opportunity to smoke when she is with Dorothy. She is a very domineering person and usually gets her way. Dorothy feels very intimidated by her. Martha can usually start Dorothy smoking again by such comments as "Oh, come on, Dorothy. This is the only chance I get to smoke and I hate to do it alone" or "Here, take one of these. No one will ever know. Besides, you've had a tough day and a smoke will calm you down." After constant persuasion of this nature Dorothy begins to think "Maybe she's right. I need something to calm my nerves" or "Oh, well, I hate to disappoint her. After all, she is my best friend." Since Dorothy does not want to avoid all contacts with Martha she must establish the following goals:

1. Discuss with Martha her influence on Dorothy's smoking behavior.
2. Learn to be more assertive with Martha and stand up for her rights as a nonsmoker.
3. Learn to control her negative thinking and rationalizations when she's with Martha.

Now, these goals are a bit more difficult to accomplish than those listed for Hi-Pac #1. The reason is that they require the development of new interpersonal and cognitive self-control skills. To be successful Dorothy must learn how to deal with Martha effectively and how to control her own thought processes. In fact, many of the goals you set as the result of your personal behavioral analysis will require that you learn new skills that will undoubtedly have a dramatic impact on your life. In an attempt to control her smoking Dorothy may have to become more assertive, learn how to relax, learn how to restructure her thought patterns, and learn how to be much more physically active. Changes in these areas may require significant modifications in her life style which may lead not only to permanent control of her smoking habit but also to a more satisfying day-to-day existence.

All you should be concerned about in this chapter is the establishment of behavioral goals based upon careful self-observation. Don't worry about exactly how you'll be achieving these goals as yet. Subsequent chapters will teach you the skills required.

Ultimate Long-Term Goal—Abstinence versus Moderation

One basic question regarding habit patterns is whether it is best to quit completely (to be totally abstinent) or to cut down on consumption and learn to smoke, drink, or eat in moderation. Certainly you cannot live without food. You can, however, decide to refrain totally from certain kinds of food. Let's take bread, for example. Some people can learn to eat rolls and bread in moderation. They can eat one roll and leave it at that. For others, especially those who have been overweight for many years, bread presents a behavioral problem. One roll leads to another and another and another. It's like the potato chip commercial that challenges the viewer with "I bet you can't eat just one!" If certain bread products or certain sweets involve behavioral problems for you, then you should probably give them up totally while dieting. Perhaps you might decide to eat bread only when someone else is around, or near the end of a meal, when your hunger is not so strong.

What about smoking? It is generally agreed that your ultimate smoking goal should be total abstinence from all cigarettes. There is still some controversy over whether you should cut down gradually until you are completely abstinent or whether to quit "cold turkey"—all at once. Again, this is an individual matter. If you have been able to quit completely before, then go ahead and do it that way again. If you have had trouble with this method, then let me suggest another way of doing it. Some research evidence suggests that people who set a target date for total abstinence from cigarettes and cut down gradually each day are the most successful at giving up smoking. The reason for the success of this method may be that by cutting down gradually and concentrating on changing your habit pattern you learn (1) what factors are influencing your smoking and (2) what procedures are effective in combating or eliminating these influences. By quitting all at once you are unable to analyze your behavior and unable to develop a new habit pattern. That is, you are not replacing the smoking habit with anything new to take its place. The gradual quitter is developing a variety of new habit-control skills which he can use permanently.

Be careful not to use this target-date method to avoid total abstinence. *Never* change the target date once it is established. Also, don't set it beyond two or three weeks. Then you should establish a schedule for yourself so that each day there is a decreasing limit on the number of cigarettes you smoke. You might decrease your consumption by 2 to 3 cigarettes a day, or 5 per day, depending on how many cigarettes you smoke and when you set your target date.

One final advantage of this gradual method is that you are less likely to experience the effects of nicotine withdrawal. The tension, nervousness, and irritability that are associated with abrupt termination of smoking are almost intolerable for some people. They may be so upsetting that you begin smoking to avoid them. Gradual withdrawal eliminates this problem almost completely. That is not to say that you still won't get cravings to smoke. With this gradual procedure, however, urges are more likely to be psychological rather than physical in nature. There are those of you who might say that when you've tried to quit smoking in the past you managed to cut down to about ten cigarettes, but you can't seem to get below that level. Unfortunately, this is quite common, but I would suggest that you continue to try to reduce your smoking to zero. If you continue to fail, then you may decide to reevaluate your goal so that ten cigarettes per day becomes your ultimate achievable goal. Be certain that you have implemented all of the procedures in this book before you make your final decision. Sometimes smoking in moderation and maintaining that moderation can be much more difficult than complete abstinence. Ten cigarettes can lead to 11, then 12, then 13, and so on. Ultimately, however, smoking 10 cigarettes per day is much better than 20 or 30 or 50. Reduction in consumption is better than no reduction at all. In fact, several colleagues of mine and I conducted a smoking study recently and found a surprising number of people who could be labeled as light smokers or controlled smokers. These people rarely smoked more than ten cigarettes on any one day, and usually smoked a lot less. On many days they simply did not smoke at all or had only one or two cigarettes. For the most part their smoking was specific to particular situations, such as parties and social gatherings. Just remember, however, that controlled, moderate smoking may require much more vigilance and much more consistent habit control than abstinence. So consider this goal carefully and only after attempting complete abstinence several times. You may also find that after a few weeks of moderate smoking you are able to give it up completely with little difficulty. In essence, you must experiment and determine what works best for *you*.

Traditionally, the goal for anyone who is considered either a heavy drinker, a problem drinker, or an alcoholic has been total and complete abstinence, with no exceptions. In fact this opinion is held very strongly by members of Alcoholics Anonymous. At the outset let me say that the self-help methods described in this book are aimed primarily at what I call the heavy social drinker. This is an individual who has not suffered severe social, emotional, occupational, marital or health problems as the result of his drinking. He may be just beginning to realize that he is drinking too much, and is trying to prevent these severe consequences from occurring. This is not to say that the principles described here cannot be used by persons labeled alcoholics. Indeed, a colleague of mine, Dr. Marie Mastria, and I recently wrote a book designed for alcoholism counselors to use with clients. That book described some of the same procedures used here. However, a person who has experienced significant problems because of chronic alcohol abuse is in need of professional help and would need more than this self-help book has to offer. Most chronic alcohol abusers probably must learn to live without alcohol. Recent research, however, is investigating the possibility that some chronic alcohol abusers may be able to learn to drink in a controlled, moderate manner. It has not as yet been determined which types of alcoholics can learn to moderate their drinking and which must be totally abstinent. While this very controversial research continues, most alcoholism treatment programs use total abstinence as the sole treatment goal.

The heavy drinker at whom this book is aimed should be able to achieve a goal of moderate, controlled drinking. The specifics of this goal in terms of amount and frequency of drinking are described in detail in Chapter 7. Generally, I would suggest a goal of moderate, controlled drinking for a heavy drinker who is concerned about his drinking. However, if you are unable to consistently moderate your drinking using these behavioral principles, you may have more of a drinking problem than you thought. In that case I would strongly advise you to seek advice from an alcoholism agency or to consider total abstinence.

Attitudes

An important phenomenon related to your choice of a smoking, eating, or drinking goal is known as *loss of control*. In a sense this involves (1) your attitudes about your ability to control your habit and (2) the expectations you have about how cigarettes, food, or alcohol will affect you. One of the most prevalent counterproductive expectations of people who smoke, overeat, or overdrink is referred to as the "loss of control" hypothesis. "Loss of control" thinking assumes that once you consume even a small amount of a cigarette, an alcoholic beverage, or a high-calorie food, you are doomed to continue consumption in spite of your best efforts. This notion implies that continued consumption is the response to an irresistible impulse over which a person has no control. Thus people say, "I don't know what came over me. Just one puff of that cigarette triggered some craving in me and I just had to have more."

Recent research evidence indicates that the "loss of control" phenomenon is *not* a *true* phenomenon in the physiological sense. That is, one drink of an alcoholic beverage or one piece of chocolate cake does not trigger some biochemical mechanism in you that leads to loss of control. The important factor in loss of control is whether or not you *believe* you have no control over your favorite substance once you begin to consume just a bit of it. If your expectation is that you will go on a binge after one drink, then you will go on a binge after one drink. Belief in the "loss of control" notion can keep you from effectively changing your habit pattern. It may also help you to rationalize continued substance abuse and avoid personal responsibility for change.

Another attitude that may make it more difficult for you to accomplish your goals is related to the *consequences* of smoking, drinking, and overeating. When you eat or drink or light up a cigarette, is it your expectation that the outcome of that behavior will be mostly positive or mostly negative? More likely than not you expect positive effects. You might say to yourself, "Drinking this beer will make me more sociable" or "A cigarette will calm me down" or "I'll feel less· depressed if I eat." Food in and of itself has no power to alleviate depression. However, your belief that it does increases the likelihood that you will continue to overeat when depressed. Depending on your past experiences, your attitudes may continue to influence your behavior in spite of concrete evidence to the contrary. For example, Dr. Peter Nathan, of Rutgers University, has found that alcohol consumption among problem drinkers leads to *increased* anxiety and depression even though drinkers expect to feel *more* relaxed after consumption.

Finally, your general attitudes toward the use and abuse of food, tobacco, and alcohol may be related to the eventual control you exert over your habit. Favorable attitudes toward the use of substances to make you feel better or enable you to enjoy life more fully are likely to maintain your habit pattern. Unfortunately, we are all constantly bombarded with advertisements that promise instant peace of mind by smoking or instant charisma by downing a couple of beers. You are encouraged not to resist hunger, because Brand X Candy will give you instant energy!

Expectations, beliefs, and attitudes play a big part in successful or unsuccessful habit control. You must be prepared to evaluate and modify your attitudes prior to embarking on a behavior-change program. No matter what others tell you or what you see on television you must believe that:

1. You *can* control your consumption patterns even after you've had just one bite, sip, or puff.
2. In the long run, the consequences of overconsumption are much more negative than positive.
3. Abuse of food, tobacco, and alcohol is inherently bad and keeps you dependent on external sources of gratification. True personal fulfillment can come only from within yourself and through the enjoyment of nonsubstance-oriented activities that enable you to "keep your mouth shut."

Read each of these new beliefs over very carefully. Say them to yourself at least once a day. Brainwash yourself into really believing these and you will have a much easier time of habit control. I think you'll find that the adoption of these beliefs will lead to the development of a new philosophy in which you examine your priorities and in which tobacco, food, or alcohol becomes essentially unimportant.

CHAPTER FOUR

Breaking Your Bad Habits

Most people think of self-control as an inner strength, a power of the will. Defined in this way self-control is a trait, a personal characteristic that you either have or don't have. There's no in-between. For example, an overeater is often described as having *no willpower*. Can someone really have absolutely no willpower? No self-control at all? I say definitely "No!"

If you think of self-control in all-or-none terms, you're walking on thin ice. If you truly believe, even for a minute, that you really lack self-control, you'll be defeated before you begin. You will use this supposed lack of willpower as an excuse for overindulgence.

Let me begin by modifying your ideas about willpower. Keep in mind that

1. Everybody, *including you,* has self-control.
2. With just a little effort you can learn to develop your self-control more fully.
3. Self-control refers to actions, not to inner strength.

You *must* believe in these three characteristics of self-control in order to succeed. *Forget your past failures.* This is a new system, remember?

First of all, as I have said, self-control is *not* an all-or-none personality trait. Everybody has self-control to a degree; some people have simply developed it and practiced it more fully. Self-control is a skill that you can build up through appropriate effort and practice. Most overeaters and heavy smokers and drinkers completely overlook episodes of their own self-control. When clients in my weekly weight-control clinic discuss their progress since the previous session, they invariably recount the episodes in which they have succumbed to temptation. In fact, the first fifteen minutes of each session sounds like group confession. Clients seem to be trying to outdo one another in reciting their "sins." When I examine each person's eating pattern for the week, there are numerous situations in which the opportunity to overeat presented itself, but the dieter resisted. For every episode of cheating there are at least a half dozen occasions demonstrating self-control. No mention is ever made by clients of their successes. They focus exclusively on failures. While this may seem to be very strange or self-defeating behavior, it is quite understandable in light of our society's view of dieting. That is, much too much emphasis is placed on weight loss in and of itself. When little thought is given to permanent change in habits, *positive* behavior patterns are overlooked.

Another reason for overemphasizing failure is that appropriate behavior, behavior that is idealized by our society, is *expected* to occur. Self-control is taken for granted because people are *supposed to* delay gratification of their desires. Let me give you an example, possibly from your own childhood. What do many parents do when their child is behaving well? The answer is "Nothing." They are totally unresponsive; the message they are conveying is, "I expect you to act this way, and you deserve no credit for doing what you're supposed to do." On the other hand, how do parents respond to misconduct? Usually they act quickly and decisively, leaving the impression that misbehavior is terrible and that he should feel guilty about his lack of self-control. Now, discipline is absolutely necessary, but why punish misconduct and fail to reward everyday good behavior? The moral of the story is that you may have been trained to ignore your "good" behavior, your self-control. I'm simply telling you that it's impression that misbehavior is terrible and that the child should Give yourself credit where credit is due.

Another characteristic of self-control is that it varies from one situation to another. You may have excellent self-control under one set of circumstances but be a pushover in a different situation. You may find when you're with other people you can resist smoking a cigarette with no difficulty; however, when you're alone, after a rough day, your willpower suddenly disappears.

Think of willpower as *self-management* rather than self-control. Think of it as managing your habit just as you'd manage a business. In this sense, self-control refers to a set of management skills, specific behaviors that decrease the chances of your smoking, overeating, or overdrinking. Self-management involves planning ahead. By planning weekly menus ahead of time you are demonstrating self-control over eating behavior. By planning to avoid a route to your office that takes you right past a cigarette machine every day, you're exhibiting self-control in regard to smoking. You might not consider such planning to be self-control, but it certainly is. Perhaps you think of self-control as standing in front of the cigarette machine arguing with yourself about whether to buy a pack or not, and convincing yourself not to. This is *one* form of self-control, primarily cognitive control. But control-

ling behavior on the spot is only a small part of managing
your behavior.

Self-Observation

In Chapter 3, I described the importance of self-observation
to determine what influences your habits. Observing your behavior can also serve as a self-control technique, a simple way
to begin to reduce your consumption. When you write down
the number of cigarettes, alcoholic beverages, or calories you
consume each day, you'll automatically consume less. Self-
monitoring simply makes you more aware of your habit. It
provides you with continuous feedback on how much you
consume, how frequently you consume, and under what circumstances you consume. Such feedback is an essential element of behavior change. You may be totally unaware of
exactly how much you consume each day and even actively
avoid finding out. Overeaters avoid scales and mirrors. Smokers lose track of their packs of cigarettes and end up smoking
from several different packs. Heavy drinkers rarely use shot
glasses to measure the liquor for their drinks. They just pour
from the bottle an amount that could vary from 1 to 4 ounces.

Typically, self-monitoring reduces your consumption to a
lower level and then seems to lose its impact. For example,
suppose you smoke on the average 40 cigarettes a day. Once
you begin to make notes on your smoking behavior your
consumption is likely to drop to 30–35 cigarettes per day and
then level off. As long as you make your daily self-observations, you'll be able to maintain this level.

In addition to your daily entries, keep a master graph that
shows your consumption pattern over time. Each day add up
the number of calories you consume, and you'll actually see

how self-monitoring affects your behavior. You'll see a drop in the first few days and then a leveling-off phase. Your daily caloric intake will stabilize at this new, lower level. Looking at the graph each day will provide the extra motivation you need from time to time. The graph can indicate slight variations and decreases in consumption that perhaps you were not aware of.

Self-observation alone will not lead to drastic, permanent behavior change. However, it can provide quick changes right at the beginning, which will give you a big boost of encouragement.

When monitoring your habits

1. Write down *every* episode of consumption.
2. Keep a note pad or index card with you at all times.
3. Record each episode of consumption *before* rather than after it occurs.

This latter point is a simple but important one. If you get ready to have a snack and have to write down how many calories you are about to consume, you probably won't eat as much. You'll be more aware of what you're eating and that you're adding another point on your graph. If you monitor your behavior *after* it occurs, it may influence your next episode of consumption, but it's too late to influence the one that just occurred. Remember, make your entry *before* each cigarette, drink, or snack, not *after*.

Controlling the Impact of Temptations
One unfortunate characteristic of overconsumers is that they are overly sensitive to the sight, smell, and taste of food,

alcohol, or tobacco. In a sense, their "stimulation tolerance level" is too low. The mere sight of food, alcohol, or cigarettes stimulates cravings and the desire to consume. An obese person may eat, not because of hunger but because a dozen chocolate chip cookies are sitting on the kitchen counter. The reason for eating a cookie under these circumstances is the same reason given for climbing a mountain—because it's there. *Remember, the more visible and available food, cigarettes, and alcohol are, the more likely you are to consume them.*

Dr. William Johnson conducted an interesting study at the University of Rochester a few years ago to show just how important the mere sight of food can be in triggering overweight people to eat. He found that obese people were much more motivated to obtain sandwiches wrapped in clear plastic wrap than those wrapped in nontransparent paper. When they could see the food they were more likely to eat it. Even though they knew that the packages wrapped in opaque paper were similar to the sandwiches in plastic wrapping, they were less motivated to eat them, because they were not *visible.* An even more interesting finding is that people who are not overweight are not as influenced by the mere sight of food.

There is obviously something different about overweight individuals that makes them more susceptible to visual cues. Only recently have scientists begun to study exactly what goes on in the body when an overweight individual sees food. Eating has been associated with certain visual stimuli so many times that the mere sight of food triggers a physiological reaction similar to one that occurs when you are actually eating. It's a minireaction, which whets your appetite by giving you a sampling of what it will feel like if you eat the food. This occurs because of a simple conditioning process similar to that observed in Pavlov's dog. Ivan Pavlov, a Russian physiologist performing research on glandular secretions at the turn of the century, conducted a simple but now classic study of how this process occurs. A hungry dog was placed in a harness to prevent him from moving. Saliva from his salivary glands was measured through a tube inserted in the dog's cheek and running into a glass container. Visual stimuli were presented to the dog to measure his reactions. For example, when the dog was shown powdered food he began to salivate. When a tone was sounded, nothing happened. To condition the dog, Pavlov sounded a tone and then immediately presented the food. This tone ⟶ food sequence was presented over and over again until the dog salivated to the tone alone, without the food being present. The dog learned to respond to a noise as if the food were present.

Overweight individuals are conditioned in the same way. Every time you look at and think about a certain food before you eat it, you're conditioning yourself to react physically to the *sight* and *thought* of food alone. Pictures of food provoke the same reaction. As I'll discuss later in this chapter, various factors in your eating environment can begin to trigger your appetite through this same conditioning process.

Recent biochemical research supports this conditioning concept by demonstrating that actual physiological changes occur in overweight people merely as a consequence of looking at desirable foods. In one study of obese adolescents it was observed that the sight of certain food resulted in increased insulin flow. This is exactly what happens when you eat sweets or starches. These foods raise your blood sugar level and your body uses insulin to readjust this level. Under conditions in which you aren't eating, insulin flow would lower your blood sugar level. Decreased blood sugar level frequently, but not always, makes you feel hungry. All of this means that if you are overweight, the mere sight of food will make you hungry. Your craving for food when you see it may indeed be a true physiological hunger and not just psychological.

Heavy smokers and heavy drinkers have a similar problem. While there has been less research on this issue with smokers and drinkers, I believe that the same factors operate in these addictions. For example, when problem drinkers are exposed to such stimuli as bottles of liquor or the sounds of a bar, their muscle tension automatically increases. Drinkers who are taught to control this muscle tension are much better able to withstand the sights and sounds of alcohol and alcohol-related activities and to control cravings to drink. *You must learn to control your mind and your body in order to conquer visual temptation!*

This extreme reactivity to visual cues is a particular problem because of the tremendous advertising emphasis on food, cigarettes, and alcohol in our society. A quick survey of newspapers, magazines, and television provides a good example. We are constantly bombarded with pictures of all the things we're trying to avoid. Almost every magazine you pick up is filled with page after page of vividly colored Danish pastries, macaroni, Bloody Marys, and the newest low-tar and -nicotine cigarette. Since you are more sensitive to these images, your cravings will be constantly stimulated—almost every day.

What can you do about your responsiveness to external cues? The first technique of self-control is to decrease the sensory impact of the substance you are most likely to consume. At the beginning of your habit-control plan of action

1. Remove all unnecessary food, cigarettes, or alcohol from your house.
2. Keep food and alcohol supplies low.
3. Keep desirable substances in inaccessible locations.
4. Keep substances out of sight by covering them or storing them in cabinets.

If you are quitting smoking completely, for example, simply remove all cigarettes from your house, office, car, or wherever else you keep them. Throw out or give away every cigarette you have. If you are cutting down your consumption but not abstaining, keep your supplies low. Similarly, keep alcoholic supplies to a minimum. Avoid the temptation to buy large quantities to save money. You may spend less per ounce by buying a gallon of Bourbon instead of a pint, but you're likely to drink more that way too. I have often heard heavy drinkers say, "But I *have* to keep a lot of booze around for friends who drop by." If this statement sounds to you like a good excuse for insuring a steady supply of liquor for someone who drinks too much, you're well on your way to controlling your habits. If the statement sounds reasonable and rational, you still have a long way to go in your thinking.

When company is expected or when you're having a party, buy liquor supplies on the day of the party. If excess liquor is left over, take it back for a refund (many liquor stores will allow this if you arrange for it ahead of time) or give it away to close friends and relatives. Keep liquor stored down in the basement or in a cabinet that's difficult to reach. If you keep beer in the refrigerator, store it behind other items so it's not staring you in the face every time you open the door. Also, don't buy beer in bottles. If you can see the beer itself through the container you will be stimulated to drink it.

Remember, the old adage "Out of sight, out of mind" is even more true for you than for other people. You *must* keep alcohol out of sight and difficult to get to. If you have to go to a hard-to-get-at location in the basement to get a bottle of gin to make a drink, you're more likely to forget the whole thing and have a soft drink instead. If you do decide to have a drink, replace the bottle in its out-of-the-way storage location *immediately* after fixing the drink. Yes, I know it's inconvenient, but do it anyway. Remember, you're indulging in a little planned willpower. If the bottle is not readily available, you're less likely to fix a second drink.

Food is a slightly different matter. You certainly must keep *some* food in your kitchen. You may, however, decide to keep certain foods out of your house. Snack foods are a good example. After a dieter confesses to me that he or she broke down at midnight and ate a whole cherry pie, I often ask, "Why did you have the pie around in the first place?" Certain "dangerous" foods, such as bread or rolls, can be stored in out-of-the-way cabinets. If sweets or snacks are available for others in your family, keep them inaccessible to you. If you have to stare at the leftovers of a pecan pie every time you open the refrigerator for your cottage cheese, you've had it. Maybe not right away, but sooner or later the sight of that pie will affect you. Why make it harder for yourself to control your eating habit?

A useful technique is to make leftovers less visible by covering them with opaque wrap such as aluminum foil, as opposed to a clear plastic or paper wrap. Can you imagine anything more unappetizing when you open the refrigerator than the blinding glare of row upon row of aluminum-covered containers? Of course not. And food companies know this too. Many foods are packaged with clear wrap to entice you into buying them. Why not make it a challenge to beat these experts at their own game? Anyway, the next time you're in the grocery store, accept the challenge head on. Be aware of the gimmicks used to make foods look more appetizing. Then use the thought-control techniques described in Chapter 6.

Pavlov's Dog in Reverse

In learning to cope with the visual aspects of temptation you must follow a two-stage process. Stage 1 involves the avoidance of as many of the visual cues associated with your preferred substance as I have just described. This stage should be in effect for at least 30 days, and possibly longer, especially for dieters who must lose a significant amount of weight. Because we are all constantly surrounded by food, tobacco, and alcohol through our interactions with others, you must eventually learn to adjust to the visual presence of these substances. This is when Stage 2 begins. Remember Pavlov's experiment? Well, that is one way in which you became over-reactive to visual stimuli. There is also a reverse conditioning procedure known as *extinction* which you can use to make yourself less responsive to these cues. Again, the process is rather simple. Pavlov found that after the dog had been conditioned to salivate to the sound of the tone, if he sounded the tone over and over again without the food, the dog would salivate less and less. Eventually the dog stopped salivating completely in response to the tone. This means that if you fail to eat when you are repeatedly exposed to visual stimuli associated with eating, you will no longer respond as strongly to these stimuli. In fact, you would be retraining your body and desensitizing yourself.

You must be very careful and proceed with this extinction technique cautiously. If you go too fast you could precipitate strong cravings. Under such circumstances it's easy to feel discouraged by discovering that your responsiveness to the mere sight of alcohol, cigarettes, or food is still strong.

I'll describe how to modify your reactions to what you see by telling you about Kevin. Kevin is a thirty-four-year-old bachelor who is an associate professor of economics at a Midwestern university. He is a studious type who enjoys his work, and because of his exceptional research and teaching abilities, is being considered for a full professorship. Physically, Kevin has a rather "lean and hungry" look, so weight control is *not* one of his problems. He drinks alcohol in moderation and could really take it or leave it. However, he is completely and totally addicted to cigarette smoking. Kevin began experimenting with cigarettes at the early age of thirteen and was smoking regularly by age sixteen. Since graduating from college he has smoked two to three packs of cigarettes every day of his life. Kevin is well aware of the health hazards of smoking, but it's been difficult for him to quit. This time he's determined to make it.

For one month he completely avoids cigarettes. The first week is really rough and Kevin feels as though he's going crazy. He's irritable, jumpy, and generally miserable. Then he begins to experience many of the positive effects of not smoking. He can breathe more deeply and play tennis longer without huffing and puffing. He even beats Dennis, a long-standing tennis rival who has never lost to him. Food tastes better.

As part of his personal antismoking campaign Kevin avoids the sight of cigarettes and anything related to them. His plan involves

1. Removing all cigarettes from his apartment and automobile.
2. Removing all ashtrays from his office, apartment, and car. (That's right! He even took the ashtray and lighter out of his car.)
3. Avoiding cigarette displays in grocery stores and drug stores.
4. Consciously looking away from cigarette machines, highway billboards advertising cigarettes, and other stimulants to his smoking habit.
5. Temporarily avoiding heavy-smoking friends.
6. Temporarily avoiding cocktail parties and other social gatherings at which many people would be smoking.

After six weeks of this regime Kevin was ready to desensitize himself to the sights of cigarettes. As a first step he chose a time of day when the likelihood of smoking was slim. This was midmorning, from about 10:30 A.M. to noon. Even when he smoked, he seldom lit up during this time. For this time interval Kevin put out ashtrays in his office, setting them out at 10:30 A.M. and putting them away at 12:00 noon. At noon each day he noted he had a craving to smoke. If such a craving occurred he rated its intensity on a scale from 0 to 10. The ashtray procedure had no detrimental effects on Kevin, so he went to the second step in his plan. He began to leave his ashtrays all day long at the office. He also replaced ashtrays at home and returned his car ashtray to its proper place. Still no problems.

Then, between 10:30 and 11:00 A.M every day he left his schedule free. He bought a pack of cigarettes, and every day for one week left it on a table in his office. He had a slight craving on one of the days, but nothing he couldn't handle. During the following week he put an opened pack of cigarettes on his desk. This resulted in one small craving the first day and none the rest of the week. During the third week Kevin took a cigarette out of the pack and placed it, along with a pack of matches, within easy reach on his desk. During the second day he experienced a strong urge to smoke while looking at the cigarette and rated his craving at 10. On the third day his craving was at 5. During the rest of the week he did not feel any more urges to smoke.

Next, Kevin attempted to modify his behavior in the morning while he was having his coffee. This had always been an especially difficult time for him to control smoking. Smoking with his morning coffee was an automatic response, a conditioned reflex. It involved no conscious thought process. At first Kevin put an ashtray next to his bed and several in the kitchen, where he drank his coffee. After a few days of no reaction he proceeded to the next step. He placed packs of cigarettes by his bedside table, on the kitchen table, and on his bathroom counter. Kevin had moderate cravings for the first three days but continued this procedure until he had gone five mornings in a row with no urges to smoke.

During the next phase Kevin placed cigarettes and matches next to his bed and in several places in the kitchen. He made it a point to look at them when he got up each day. The first day his craving for a cigarette was so strong he didn't think he'd be able to resist. The second and third were equally bad for him. He quickly decided to retreat temporarily rather than fight. He went back to just leaving closed cigarette packages around in the morning. He consciously looked at the packs every day and continued this procedure until he resumed leaving the cigarettes and matches in sight. He again had trouble on the first day, but rated his craving only at 6. His ratings for each day of the next two weeks were as follows: 6, 5, 6, 3, 0, 2, 0, 7, 0, 0, 0, 0, 0, 0. After a number of days Kevin was no longer bothered by the cigarettes.

His final step involved extending this same procedure to difficult times of the day and to different circumstances. Once this procedure was complete, he didn't go out of his way to look at cigarettes, but he didn't go out of his way to avoid them either. For example, he no longer keeps cigarettes around the house. At the same time, he is no longer bothered by seeing cigarettes or seeing people smoke.

You must keep some basic rules in mind when you use this desensitization procedure:

> _Rule 1._ Expose yourself to cigarettes or food or alcohol in a very gradual manner.
>
> _Rule 2._ Keep exposing yourself to one set of circumstances until you have gone at least 5 days (10 is better) without any urges. This is _extremely important!_
>
> _Rule 3._ If, during one step in this process, your urges are very strong for 3 or 4 days, _immediately_ stop the procedure and revert to the previous step.

Remember that you are _training_ yourself, not _testing_ yourself. The former alcoholic who keeps a bottle of whiskey around to demonstrate his willpower is asking for trouble. Training consists of a _gradual_ process during which your physical and psychological reactions to these visual cues change.

Dieters and heavy drinkers will need to desensitize themselves to restaurants and bars. After avoiding bars completely for a month or two, a heavy drinker should consciously look inside a bar. If no strong urges to drink arise, the next step involves going to a bar with a friend. This friend or relative should be a light or moderate drinker. If you are simply cutting down on your drinking, order one drink, and sip it very slowly. Pay attention to all the visual cues in the bar that might influence you.

How to Beat the Clock

The clock has a significant influence on your behavior. Eating, smoking, and drinking become associated with certain times of the day. Once you reduce your consumption you can expect to have most of your cravings at times when you used to eat, smoke, or drink. If you have developed a pattern of smoking a cigarette after each meal, then the 20- to 30-minute time interval following a meal will be a tempting one. Because of your past habit pattern, you have actually conditioned yourself to want a cigarette at certain times of the day.

The first step in overcoming this influence of the clock is to refer to the self-observations that we discussed in Chapter 3. What times of the day are you most likely to eat, drink, or smoke? Let's suppose you have the habit, as many people do, of coming home from work and settling down to two martinis, cheese, and crackers. (In fact, this is probably such a strong habit that you're cringing at the thought of giving it up.) Having determined to lose a few pounds, you decide that your early evening drinks and snacks must go. How to proceed? You *must* change your routine. As soon as you arrive home from the office, busy yourself with activities that are incompatible with eating and drinking. Better yet, have these activities planned *before* you arrive home.

For example, Tony always arrives home between 6:00 and 6:30 P.M. each evening. His job as a personnel manager is a hectic one that leaves him tense at the end of the day. He looks forward to sitting down with his wife when he gets home, having three or four beers, maybe some potato chips and dip, and discussing the events of the day. At forty-four Tony is a large, ordinarily energetic man who is definitely overweight. He has been feeling very fatigued lately, especially after work. The beers just make him sleepy, and he usually goes to bed early, soon after dinner. At the urging of his wife and his physician, he decides to change his habit patterns. Notice that I did *not* say he decides to go on a diet. As I pointed out in Chapter 1, that would not be enough to insure permanent change. Tony decides that at least for a while he has to give up his beer and snacks every evening. He also decides that in order to do this he must get involved in other activities from 6:00 to 7:00 P.M. to keep himself from drinking and eating. He makes a list of as many alternative activities as he can think of. The list includes the following:

1. Eat dinner immediately upon arriving home.
2. Take my wife and children out to dinner, shopping, or to a movie.
3. Work with my son on restoring an old car that I bought him.
4. Take an hour walk alone or with my wife.
5. Do my Royal Canadian Air Force exercises; shower and change clothes.
6. Jog for 15 minutes.
7. Talk with my wife about the day in a room other than the kitchen or family room.
8. Go for a bicycle ride with my wife.

Tony now has a choice of eight different alternative activities to fill the time when he first gets home after work. With some activities, such as eating dinner early, he will have to request the cooperation of his wife. She is more than eager to cooperate. Early each day Tony decides ahead of time what activity he'll schedule for that evening. He varies his routine to keep it from becoming too monotonous, and he finds that these changes in routine make his habit-control efforts relatively easy. He especially enjoys exercising, walking, and bicycling, and after the first week doesn't feel nearly as tired as he used to. He and his wife walk together, which gives them an opportunity to talk and share their daily experiences.

Tony's plan is an excellent one. First of all, his activities are incompatible with snacking and drinking. Second, his alternative activities are enjoyable and have positive side effects, which further lessen the chances of snacking. Because of his new emphasis on physical fitness he feels less tense and doesn't seem to need alcohol or food when he arrives home from work. By taking his wife out more and helping his son work on the car he feels closer to his family. Everybody in the family benefits. One very simple change in routine can have far-reaching effects not only on personal habit control but on life in general. It's simply a way of getting yourself out of a rut.

Through his alternative activities Tony is also teaching himself new habits. He is breaking that automatic association between 6:00 P.M. and snacking. He is establishing a new association so that more and more when he arrives home he is thinking about walking or exercising, and not eating or drinking. These new associations can become as automatic and as much of a reflex action as the old ones. As with all Personal Habit Control techniques in this book, *repetition* is the key.

And even if Tony decides to have a beer one evening, he's not locked into the habit of two or three *every* evening.

When applying this technique to your own life

1. Be aware of specific times of the day when you are most likely to overconsume.
2. Choose alternative activities that are stimulating and enjoyable.
3. Choose activities, such as exercise, that have positive side effects.
4. Choose enough activities to keep your schedule varied and interesting.
5. Plan activities at least 12 to 24 hours in advance.

Situational Control Procedure

Your plan of action must involve controlling situations associated with consumption. You must begin by establishing new associations. Look at your list of situations and activities and ask yourself, "In which ones would I be able to give up smoking, drinking, or eating the easiest?" Let's say your eating list looks like this:

> *I eat while*
> Preparing meals
> Standing in front of the refrigerator
> Watching television
> Reading
> Alone
> In bed

You may then decide that you could give up eating in bed, standing in front of the refrigerator, and while reading. That's your goal for the first week. If you are lying in bed reading a book and you feel like having a snack, either say no to the snack or go into the kitchen and eat it sitting at the kitchen table. *Do not* eat in bed or while reading, no matter what! Make a hard-and-fast rule and be stern with yourself. Deciding that you can't resist the temptation is not a good excuse. Remember, if you decide to eat, then eat, but just don't do it in bed or with a book in your hand. The same goes for eating while you're standing in the kitchen. No matter what kind of food you are eating, *do not* eat it standing up in the kitchen. You may catch yourself opening the refrigerator, taking out an apple, and while standing there, taking a large bite. This is absolutely forbidden! By doing this, even once, you're continuing the conditioned association that you're trying to break. Make yourself sit down at the table. If you have to, put a sign on the refrigerator that says, in big letters, SIT DOWN!! Or SELF-CONTROL MEANS NEVER HAVING TO STAND AND EAT! Corny, yes. But it gets the point across.

Once you're able to lie in bed, read, or stand in the kitchen several times without eating, you're ready for the next step. Choose one or two more situations on your list and give up eating then too. For example, no more eating while watching television or while preparing meals. The end result of all this should include two general rules for yourself:

1. Eat *only* in places designed for eating, such as a kitchen, dining room, or restaurant.
2. *Do not* do anything else while you are eating except eat and enjoy your meal.

You must strictly limit your consumption of food to a kitchen or dining room table. Every time you eat, whether it's a meal or snack, you should be sitting at the table, preferably in the same seat as usual. You are trying to limit the external cues that are associated with your eating and hence stimulate your appetite. After several times of not eating while watching television, for example, you'll break the pattern. After a while, only the kitchen and dining room tables will control your appetite.

It's also essential to think of eating as a pure experience in and of itself. While eating, don't do anything else, except perhaps enjoy a conversation with your eating partners. Whatever else you have to do can wait. Don't read, watch TV, browse through a magazine, or write letters.

A very successful author of my acquaintance had the habit of eating butterscotch candy while writing her novels. She developed this pattern quite innocently after her husband brought home a bag of these hard candies one day, and the pattern became so strong that she ate candy through all 344 pages of the novel she was working on. Now, that's a lot of candy, and as a result she put on a few extra pounds. To prepare for a publicity tour after the book was published she vowed to shed twenty pounds. But she wanted to get rid of this extra weight forever. She realized that her eating patterns had to change and that one of the first things to go must be butterscotch candy. However, this was no simple task. Giving up the candy was difficult enough, but she also had her superstition to contend with. Yes, that's right, superstition! Creative people are often profoundly superstitious, especially when it comes to their own creative talents. Authors, actors, and artists all fear that one day they may lose the magic ingredients that foster their creativity. Because of this artistic sensitivity they develop superstitions about anything associated with their abilities. Thus the burning question and deep concern of my author friend was, "Will I still be able to write as well *without* butterscotch candy?" Intellectually, she realized that such a question was silly, but emotionally it was a very serious consideration. Once she wrote one page without butterscotch, the next was easier, and the next easier still. The quality of her writing was as good as if not better than it was before. And as page after page was completed, she completely forgot about the candy and lost all craving for it.

In the final step of situational control you must set specific rules for your consumption which limit the places and situations in which you eat, drink, or smoke. The experiences of Lou, a forty-two-year-old bank executive, will illustrate the kind of rules I'm referring to. Lou has been a heavy social drinker for about ten years. He never used to like alcohol very much, but as his career grew he found it necessary to attend more and more business social functions in which liquor flowed freely. A couple of drinks loosened him up and made him feel more congenial. His wife, Nora, fell into the same pattern. After a while they were both drinking six, seven, or even eight drinks at almost every party. At home at the end of the workday they relaxed before dinner by having three or four stiff drinks. Lou worried that his heavy drinking, especially at cocktail parties, was going to hurt his image at the bank. After all, his bank was a rather conservative one. Even a young assistant vice-president had been told recently that his handlebar mustache was not in keeping with the bank's image and either it or he would have to go.

When Lou and Nora examined their drinking patterns they realized that they did not just drink at parties and before dinner. Lou would drink beer watching television, wine with meals, and sometimes even have a couple of drinks in his workshop in back of the house. Nora occasionally had a cou-

BREAKING YOUR BAD HABITS 99

ple of glasses of wine in the afternoon, and she usually had drinks when lunching with or visiting friends. Frequently both Lou and Nora had two Bloody Marys each on Sunday morning. They agreed to limit both the quantity of their drinking and the places in which their drinking occurred. They established the following hard-and-fast rules and promised to abide by them:

> *Rule 1.* Drinking is allowed *only* between the hours of 5:00 and 11:30 P.M. Drinking at any other time is prohibited.
> *Rule 2.* Drinking is allowed *only* if someone else is present. Drinking alone is prohibited.
> *Rule 3.* Drinking is allowed *only* at home and at social gatherings. Drinking in bars or restaurants is prohibited.
> *Rule 4.* At home, drinking is allowed only in the living room while conversing with each other or with friends. Drinking in any other household location or during any other activity is prohibited.

Lou and Nora found these rules relatively easy to keep. They both decreased their drinking and felt in much better control of their lives.

Now, let's suppose you are a heavy smoker. During the first week of your "cold turkey" no-smoking efforts you must avoid as many situations and activities that have been associated with heavy consumption as possible. This might mean giving up coffee or alcoholic beverages for a week. It might involve avoiding certain rooms in the house or driving as little as possible or not talking on the telephone. Simultaneously, you should spend as much time as possible in situations and activities that have not been associated with smoking. You might have to take a lot of showers, jog more, go to the movies, visit friends who disapprove of smoking, or go to restaurants with no-smoking sections. Yes, this involves drastic changes in your life style for at least a week. But you must be prepared to make these changes and not allow anything to get in your way. This is why it's very important to plan your quitting day ahead of time.

After a seven- to ten-day period of avoidance, it's time to gradually take part again in the activities and reappear in the places that are more likely to trigger smoking. Arrange your list of situations in a hierarchy, with ones that are likely to be most difficult for you at the top and those in which you could more easily refrain from smoking at the bottom. Gradually begin by exposing yourself to the situations near the bottom of the list and work your way up to the top. You'll find that the more often you endure a particular circumstance without smoking, the easier it becomes. After drinking several cups of coffee without smoking, you'll gradually learn to cope with this situation. Coffee drinking will gradually lose its association with cigarettes. By simply avoiding coffee drinking, you're not teaching yourself to respond differently.

You can also change certain conditions relating to your former activities. For example, you may experience less of a desire to smoke if you drink your morning coffee in a room other than the usual one. If drinking alcohol with lunch is the problem, you can have lunch brought into the office, eat at a restaurant that doesn't serve alcohol, or, if possible, go home for lunch every once in a while.

You can also lessen the sharpness of a craving by providing your mouth or hands with an alternative to smoking or drinking alcohol. Busy hands and mouths are happy hands and mouths. Try fiddling with a pencil instead of smoking a cigarette while talking on the telephone. Chew gum instead of smoking while watching television. Some people even find nicotine substitute gum (available at most drugstores) helpful as an alternative and as a way of coping with the nicotine withdrawal syndrome. If you're refraining from alcohol, keep a glass of water, club soda, or Perrier water in your hand. Drink one of these, with a twist of lime or lemon, instead of a cocktail when you're at a party or when you get home from work.

Use your imagination to think of more alternatives. Try one of the following activities to keep your hands occupied:

1. Doodle on a note pad.
2. Make paper airplanes.
3. Knit or sew.
4. Sketch.
5. Whittle a piece of wood.
6. Model clay.
7. Make paper-clip chains.
8. Tie different kinds of knots.
9. Work wooden hand puzzles.

Who knows? You may discover talents you were unaware of. Of course there's always the possibility of developing a new addiction. Doodling, whittling, or sketching, however, are at least healthful addictions which won't kill you, as will the ones you have now. Besides, you may end up in the *Guinness Book of World Records* for constructing the longest paper-clip chain in history!

Rewarding and Punishing Yourself

Believe it or not, your habits are also controlled by their immediate consequences, the events that occur immediately *after* you smoke, eat, or drink. For the most part, your experiences during the first few minutes after you consume a substance are very pleasurable. Otherwise you might not continue to stuff your mouth. You feel better, more relaxed perhaps, after you eat, smoke, or drink. Because you overconsume in the company of others, your behavior becomes associated with the pleasantness of interacting with friends. After a few drinks you may feel better about yourself, more confident, more self-assured, more personally powerful.

Unfortunately, habitual behaviors are more influenced by *immediate* consequences than by long-term ones. That's why your hacking cough, your hangover, and your fat have little influence on your behavior. We are all "now"-oriented, and while the ultimate effects of overconsumption make us feel bad, they don't do much to help us stop overconsuming.

To control your habit you must arrange your life so that overconsumption is punished and moderate consumption and abstinence are rewarded. Rewards and punishments can be in the form of thoughts and mental images as described in Chapter 6. External rewards frequently have more of an impact on your behavior. To implement this procedure, write down a list of as many activities as possible that you find pleasurable or satisfying. Your list might look like this:

> Reading mystery novels
> Solving crossword puzzles
> Listening to classical music
> Watching football on television

Going to the movies
Playing handball
Buying new clothes
Talking on the telephone

Now, before you can reward or punish yourself with these activities you must set a goal for yourself each day. If you are controlling your weight, your daily goals might consist of (1) limiting your consumption of food to 1,000 calories, and (2) eating only three meals, with no snacks in between. Your daily smoking goal might be to refrain totally from cigarettes. Your drinking goal might be to limit yourself to two drinks per day.

Once you've established a daily goal, choose any one of the pleasurable activities on your list. Let's suppose you choose reading the mystery novel you've been enjoying so much. Starting tomorrow, make a deal with yourself to read your book *only*—and I really mean *only*—if you have attained your goal for that day. If you've stuck to your diet, then reward yourself with the opportunity to read. However, if you've cheated, if you've had even a snack between meals, punish your behavior by withholding the reward. That's right! Tell yourself you cannot read the book. Now, that's self-control—being in charge of disciplining yourself.

Each day you should choose a different reward or a combination of rewards. Don't be easy on yourself. Choose activities that you really enjoy, and take them up only if you've controlled your habit. If you have attained your goal every day during the week, give yourself a grand reward at the end of the week. Buy something frivolous for yourself. Do something enjoyable that you've been meaning to do but have been postponing. Go on a skiing weekend, for example.

You must be consistent and strict with yourself in granting these rewards. Don't make excuses. For example, after you've smoked a cigarette, *do not* say, "Oh, well, I've learned my lesson. Besides, this is a once-in-a-lifetime fight on TV tonight. I just can't miss it." You can, if you want to learn to develop self-control!

One way to insure that you abide by all the rules you've set for your behavior is to make your reward plan public. Let your family and/or close friends know what you're up to. Better yet, prepare a written statement of your proposed self-reward system and give a copy to selected people. Then, if you don't follow through with your plan, everyone will know about it.

Behavioral Contracts

A formal written statement of your intent to reward yourself for controlling your habit is called a *behavioral contract*. Actually, it's just like a business contract, only you're making it with yourself. It's also possible, and in many cases preferable, to negotiate a behavioral contract with another person. Again, this insures that your reward-and-punishment system will be implemented.

Contracts can be beneficial to two people at the same time, especially if each one is giving up a habit. Phil and Alice are a married couple with no children. They live in New York City, where Phil is a computer programmer and Alice manages a photography shop. Phil is thirty-six years old and about twenty-five pounds overweight. He loves sweets and, in addition to eating desserts, makes nightly visits to an ice cream parlor located near their home. He always orders a butterscotch sundae with extra whipped cream. Alice is thirty-three and has little trouble watching her weight. She's been after Phil to lose a few pounds for months. He's been encouraging her to quit smoking. She smokes about a pack a day, a habit that Phil detests. He can't stand the smell of cigarette smoke and stale ashes drive him crazy. One day they agree to do something about their habits through the use of a mutual behavioral contract.

There are two things you should know about Phil and Alice which will be important as we discuss their use of a self-reward system. First, both are liberal Democrats who pride themselves on being very concerned and active in the area of human rights. Second, both are rather frugal individuals who are very careful to use money wisely.

After a lengthy discussion Phil and Alice agree on behavioral contracts. Alice's contract follows:

Behavioral Contract

1. Alice agrees to write ten checks for $20 each and give them to Phil.
2. Each will be made out to the Ku Klux Klan.
3. For each consecutive three-day period that Alice refrains from smoking, Phil will tear up one $20 check in Alice's presence.
4. If Alice smokes during any three-day period, Phil will immediately send a $20 check as a contribution from Alice to the Ku Klux Klan.
5. If Alice smokes and forfeits a $20 check, a new three-day time period will begin immediately.
6. Forfeiture of a $20 check will be determined by Phil's observation of Alice's smoking, Alice's reporting to Phil that she smoked, or reports to Phil from several selected friends and coworkers.

     7. This contract shall be posted in a conspicuous place at Alice's office and at home.

Phil's contract is similar except that his goal is to eat no more than 1,200 calories per day and to lose at least one pound per week. His $20 checks are to be made out to the John Birch Society.

How's that for self-control? Phil and Alice have arranged self-control contracts they're sure they won't break. And that's the idea! *Not* to break the contract! Each time Alice smokes or Phil goes off his diet, they'll not only be losing $20 but also contributing to organizations to which they are vehemently opposed.

After all checks are either torn up or sent off as contributions, Phil and Alice can renegotiate their contracts. Both may feel that they have gained enough habit control by the end of the contract time so that they no longer need the agreements. Now they can switch to mental rewards (see Chapter 6) or to less severe consequences, such as restrictions on golf or tennis activities.

CHAPTER FIVE

—— Personal Relaxation Training

Let's examine some of the things that happen when you change your habits. Many effects of Personal Habit Control, both immediate and long-term, are positive. You *feel* better, possibly *look* better, and certainly *live longer*. If you're a smoker, food tastes better, your breath smells better, you breathe more easily, you have a sense of personal accomplishment, and you'll live a longer and healthier life.

Unfortunately, you've gotten so accustomed to having your habit around, you're likely to mourn it when its gone. That's right! You may actually grieve for it as if you've lost someone close to you. After all, your old habit provided you with a certain amount—perhaps a *significant* amount—of pleasure and satisfaction. Also, much of your time each day was spent practicing your habit. When the habit is removed, a large piece of your total life will also be removed. You'll feel a void. You'll not only have extra time to fill but you'll experience less pleasure in your life. In fact, many people experience a mild depression after changing their habit patterns. This is by no means inevitable, so don't let me discourage or upset you. Just be wary of adopting the mistaken notion that once you overcome your old habits everything in your life will be absolutely wonderful.

Keep in mind that

Changing your habits will *not* necessarily make you totally and permanently happy.

Both positive *and* negative effects may result from changing your habits.

While many positive benefits occur *automatically* when you change habits, other benefits require specific effort from you to coax them along.

Dr. Leonard Epstein, of the University of Pittsburgh, and Dr. John Martin, of the University of Mississippi, recently evaluated the side effects of a weight-control treatment program. The patients were all overweight college students who attended a weekly class in which they learned strategies for changing their eating patterns. The effects of the program on weight and health were very positive. Not only did patients lose significant amounts of weight but blood-pressure values decreased substantially. One patient, for example, reduced her blood pressure from 148/100 to 133/75 after weight loss. However, no changes occurred in the social lives of the dieters. You might expect that after losing weight an individual would feel more sociable and less self-conscious. You might expect him or her to interact more with other people. This is not necessarily true. Social interaction requires initiation on your part. People aren't going to flock to you simply because you've given up an old habit.

The way to cope with the possibility of negative side effects is to develop a variety of alternative activities to serve as substitutes for smoking, eating, or drinking. First and foremost, alternative activities must be pleasurable. Since you're losing a familiar pleasure by modifying your habit, you *must* have a specific replacement to make up for the loss. Such activities as reading, walking, bicycling, dancing, listening to music, sewing, exercising, or developing a specific hobby are good replacements. Second, you must be able to use your alternative at times when you are most likely to smoke, eat, or drink. The activity must be readily available. Going on a ski weekend might be extremely pleasurable, but it could not serve as an immediate substitute for substance abuse. Such alternatives as exercising, painting, sculpturing, letter writing, or stamp collecting would be more practical.

In searching for alternatives, consider the antecedent events that precipitate your habit. Think back to your self-assessment, as suggested in Chapter 3, and consider the circumstances that immediately precede your overconsumption. These might include

> Boredom
> Feeling tense and restless
> Sunday afternoon and evening
> Coming home from work
> Being home alone
> Fatigue

Now, let's suppose you usually smoke a great deal on Sunday afternoon when you feel bored and restless. Think of this as a problem situation to which you must come up with several solutions. As you consider various alternatives to smoking, ask yourself these questions about each:

1. Will this activity give me pleasure?
2. Will this activity be readily available with minimal preplanning involved?
3. Will this activity relieve my boredom and restlessness?
4. Will this activity be healthful for me?

Actually, you can consider smoking as one response to your problem situation. Let's answer the above questions with smoking as the activity in question. In answer to the first three questions above, smoking will certainly give you pleasure, it's readily accessible, and it is likely, at least temporarily, to relieve your boredom and restlessness. However, in response to Question 4 you must reply, "No." Smoking is definitely not healthful, and thus you must discard it as a solution. As you can see, your bad habits can at times be viewed as coping mechanisms that function to improve your state of affairs, at least temporarily. Unfortunately, these effects are short-lived and have serious negative side effects.

The most practical solution is to develop a list of *various* activities that can distract you. These might include walking, writing, painting, or reading. These are all healthful alternatives that are close at hand.

Let me go into some detail on the use of two types of alternatives that I consider to be your best choices. They include (1) relaxation and (2) recreational activities.

Personal Relaxation Training

Total physical and mental relaxation is one of the most useful alternatives to smoking, drinking, and overeating available to you. The ability to relax can help you in several ways. First, relaxation can alleviate tension and anxiety, which often lead to "emotional overconsumption," or binges. Instead of eating, smoking, or drinking when you're tense, simply relax. Then you won't need to overconsume, since you will have found a better solution to the precipitating event. Unfortunately, our society tends to foster the abuse of substances to relieve anxiety. Perhaps your parents were in the habit of giving you candy or cookies to make you feel better when you were upset. Conditioning of eating patterns begins very early in life. The association between unhappiness and eating is very strong even in young children.

The mass media help to foster this notion, particularly through ads and commercials. Alcohol and nonprescription drug use are frequently portrayed as ways to relieve tension, as exciting or as "manly" behavior (particularly in the case of alcohol), and as self-rewards for jobs well done. Commercial messages show people "relaxing" by downing several beers after climbing a mountain, fighting a forest fire, or even parking a large truck in a narrow space. Other commercials encourage us to use nonprescription sedative drugs to induce relaxation or sleep. One of my favorite examples of this is a commercial that shows a young woman in a beautiful country atmosphere. The air, supposedly, is fresh, the scenery green and beautiful, and the total atmosphere is relaxing. The audience is told, however, that in spite of the relaxing surroundings the young woman shouldn't hesitate to take a pill if she has trouble sleeping. To add insult to injury, the young woman's mother shows up to say that it's perfectly okay to take sleeping pills—"Your dad takes them all the time."

Television programming, particularly in situation comedies, is also instrumental in conveying distorted attitudes about food, cigarettes, and alcohol. Recent surveys have indicated that over 80 percent of a sampling of 200 daytime and evening prime-time television programs referred in some way to the use of alcohol, which was frequently shown as a way to relieve tension and anxiety. But obviously relaxation provides a much more satisfactory answer.

In addition to relieving tension, relaxation can also help you control cravings. Cravings for food, cigarettes, or alcohol are frequently accompanied by muscle tension and feelings of intense restlessness. Craving is not merely a cognitive experience but also a physical feeling very similar to the experience of anxiety. Relaxation can actually reduce cravings and in many instances eliminate them altogether.

Learning to relax also has several side benefits. The ability to relax completely at a moment's notice gives you a feeling of control over your body. It provides you with a recognition of your "self-efficacy." Self-efficacy refers to personal power over your behavior. Dr. Albert Bandura, a distinguished psychologist at Stanford University, has postulated that feelings of self-efficacy are extremely important in determining your ability to cope with various types of personal problems in your life.

In addition, the regular practice of relaxation can actually improve your health and bodily functions. Relaxation training has been applied successfully to the treatment of high blood pressure, insomnia, headaches, ulcers, and chronic pain. I became acutely aware of the usefulness of relaxation in combating insomnia from the experience of a former patient of mine. David is a sixty-four-year-old retired automotive designer who was gradually developing a drinking problem. He used alcohol to relieve boredom and to induce sleep. Since his retirement he had had insomnia almost nightly. He found that two drinks before bedtime relaxed him enough so that he could get to sleep within fifteen minutes after going to bed. But because of a medical problem, David had had to quit drinking completely. It was not until then that he realized how dependent on alcohol he had really become. Without nightly drinks his insomnia came back in full force. Then I provided David with a cassette tape on which I had recorded my step-by-step Personal Relaxation Training procedure. On these tapes I tried to induce a feeling of relaxation by speaking in a rather slow, deep monotone. I instructed him to play the recording each evening before retiring. After a few nights the cassette worked so well that Dave fell asleep halfway through the instructions. One evening he actually fell asleep in the short pause between pushing the "Record" switch and my first word of instruction. I've been told that I speak in a very relaxed tone, but that was the first time that the anticipation of my voice had ever put anybody to sleep!

Various forms of relaxation have been popularized over the last several years. Yoga and transcendental meditation, in particular, are practiced throughout the world. Relaxation has been found to be extremely helpful in controlling addictive habit patterns. In my own practice, patients report that relaxation is one of their most successful strategies against urges to smoke, eat, or drink. Scientists such as Dr. Alan Marlatt and his colleagues at the University of Washington have begun to study the relationship between the regular practice of relaxation and addictions. For example, Dr. Marlatt compared the effects of different relaxation procedures on the alcohol consumption of social drinkers. Subjects in the experiment were taught and told to practice either (1) meditation, as described by Dr. Herbert Benson in his popular book of a few years ago, *The Relaxation Response*,* (2) a technique known as progressive muscle relaxation, which focuses on complete muscular relaxation, or (3) simply resting each day. A fourth group, the control subjects, received no specific training or instructions. He found that the daily practice of relaxation, in whatever form it was used, resulted in significantly less social drinking. People in the study who continued to practice relaxation maintained

* Herbert Benson, *The Relaxation Response*. New York: William Morrow, 1975.

lowered alcohol consumption over a considerable period of time. Relaxation training simply reduces your desire for alcohol.

Over the years I have developed my own method of teaching people to relax known as *Personal Relaxation Training.* Actually, it combines the best elements of other relaxation training techniques. The procedure is relatively simple and can be learned in about two hours' time. It is essential to progress through the training slowly in order to master each small detail. This slow approach will pay off later when you are practicing and further developing the skill of relaxation.

Personal Relaxation Training involves three distinct phases. During Phase 1 deep muscle relaxation is taught. Phase 2 emphasizes your internal bodily mechanisms, such as heart rate and respiration. In Phase 3 the focus is on mental relaxation. It is essential that you learn to relax in all three of these phases in the beginning of training. Then, after you've mastered the technique, you can emphasize whichever phase relaxes you the most. Since everybody experiences tension in a slightly different way, the techniques must be individualized according to your own responses. For example, one person will develop headaches when he's tense, while another will get a knotted, queasy feeling in his stomach. Still another will experience considerable mental anguish and worry. Some people experience all three reactions. The type of relaxation training you need depends to a great extent on which of your bodily systems becomes most disrupted when you're tense. Unfortunately, many techniques of relaxation focus only on *one* bodily system. If your anxiety is mostly in the form of muscle tension, transcendental meditation, which emphasizes cognitive relaxation, may not be effective for you. You might learn to relax using TM, but because of even slight muscle tension you won't be able to achieve deep levels of relaxation. This is exactly why I developed my own system and why I refer to it as Personal Relaxation Training. It is *personal* because it can be individualized to each person's needs and thereby be much more efficient.

Now I'll describe each phase of the relaxation process. Since it is difficult to read the description and practice the technique at the same time I suggest you read it through completely once or twice and then apply it. If you have difficulty remembering exactly what to do, ask someone in your family or a close friend to cue you in to each step as you proceed. Or you could make a tape recording, in which you serve as your own relaxation coach. I routinely make relaxation tape recordings available to patients when they are first learning this procedure.

PHASE 1: MUSCLE RELAXATION

To begin the relaxation process, seat yourself in a comfortable lounge chair or recliner. Generally the technique consists of sequentially tightening and then relaxing different muscle groups to experience maximum tension followed by gradually increasing relaxation. Each muscle group is tensed and relaxed two or three times in order to allow you to become accustomed to the bodily sensations of tight and tense muscles versus loose and relaxed muscles.

Begin by placing your arms loosely on the arms of the chair or in your lap. Now make a very tight fist with your right hand. Tighten your fist and arm muscles as if you were going to give somebody a right uppercut. When your arm muscles have reached maximum tension, relax your hand and arm very gradually. Go slowly. Concentrate on the feelings in your fingers, hand, and arm as your muscles relax. Keep letting go until your hand and arm are loose, limp, and relaxed. Proceed slowly. It should take you at least a full minute or more to go from muscle tightness to relaxation. During each step of the way concentrate on the changes occurring in your hand and arm. In addition to feeling more relaxed your muscles will also feel heavier. You may also experience a feeling of warmth in your arm. These sensations indicate that your arm is becoming *very* relaxed. When you think your arm is completely relaxed, try to take it one step further. Try to relax it and loosen it up even more. Even slight muscle tension must be eliminated.

Now go through exactly the same procedure with your other arm. Remember to proceed slowly and deliberately. Don't try to force your muscles to relax. Sometimes the harder you try, the less relaxation you'll feel. It's a little like trying to fall asleep at night. The more you consciously *try* to get to sleep, the more wide-awake you become. Just let your muscles go, let them relax naturally. Take a passive rather than an active role.

After relaxing your left hand and arm, make sure you keep both arms relaxed and in a comfortable position. Now focus your total concentration on both arms and hands. Let them relax even more. Keep relaxing them until you experience a heavy, warm, or tingling feeling in your muscles.

Next, focus your attention on your neck muscles. A great deal of tension often builds up in the neck and head regions. Keep your body straight and slowly turn your head to the right as far as possible. Feel your neck muscles stretching and tightening. Slowly turn your head so you're facing front once again. As you do so, concentrate on relaxing your neck muscles. Then turn your head to the left, stretching the muscles on the other side. Slowly turn your head back again, relaxing the muscles. Now bring your head all the way back as if you're trying to touch your upper back with the back part of your head. This movement will stretch the muscles in the front part of your neck, under your chin. Now lower your head slowly and let your neck muscles relax. Bring your chin down, touching it to the upper part of your chest. This will stretch the muscles in the back part of your neck. Slowly raise your head back into a normal position.

There are a number of small muscle groups in your face, jaws, forehead, and head that also must be tensed and relaxed. The muscles in your jaws can be tightened simply by clenching your teeth together. As you clench your teeth, place your hands on the sides of your jaws. Notice how the muscles harden as you clench. Now relax your jaws and let your mouth fall open just a slight bit. To be truly relaxed your mouth should be neither tightly shut nor wide open. Let it hang open naturally, as if you were asleep, and your jaw muscles will be completely relaxed.

Next, purse your lips in the style of an exaggerated kiss. Then let them slowly relax. Remember, with each muscle group, concentrate on the feelings in your muscles when they are completely tense and completely relaxed. The muscles around your eyes and the front part of your face can be tightened by squinting your eyes together firmly in an exaggerated fashion. Slowly release the tension. Try to imagine that all your facial muscles are sagging down.

Your forehead muscles are very important in the relaxation process. While some people have difficulty relaxing these muscles, you should be able to do it skillfully with just a little practice. Most people simply aren't accustomed to paying much attention to their forehead muscles—except, perhaps, if one is having a splitting headache. To tense these muscles, raise your eyebrows as far up as they'll go. Pretend you're being surprised and frightened at the same time. The only possible drawback in this exercise is that your spouse may enter the room just as you're doing it and may think you've flipped your lid. Just ignore any odd looks you might get and continue on. Slowly lower your eyebrows, paying particular attention to the decreasing tightness in your forehead. Now lower your eyebrows in an exaggerated frown. Pretend you're extremely worried. Feel your muscles tense as you do this. Raise your eyebrows and let your muscles relax. Keep your forehead muscles relaxing more and more even after all the tightness is gone.

In addition to the head area, your shoulders and back are very susceptible to tension. That's one reason why a back rub feels so good. Shrug your shoulders as if you're trying to touch your ears with them. Try to feel the tightness in your shoulders and upper back. Now slowly let your shoulders down, relaxing the muscles. That might feel so good you'll want to repeat it several times. Go ahead. It's perfectly okay. After you're finished with that, arch your back as if you're attempting to push both shoulders together in back of you. Then let your shoulders come back into place and hang loosely but naturally.

Before we go to your legs let's stop off at your stomach muscles for a minute. Tense your stomach muscles by pretending that someone is about to hit you there as hard as they can. Tighten that gut. Get the muscles hard. Good! Now you can let them relax.

Tighten your leg muscles by stretching your right leg out and pointing your toe out straight. This exercise will tighten the muscles in the upper part of your leg. Slowly relax the leg, concentrating on developing maximum relaxation. Repeat this same procedure with your left leg. Now go back to the right leg. Stretch it out, and bend your foot and toe back, trying to point your toe toward you. You'll really feel the tightness in your calf muscle if you're doing this right. Now slowly relax your leg and repeat the exercise with the left leg.

To relax your chest muscles, take a very deep breath. Consciously try to tighten your chest muscles after you have inhaled as much air as you can. Slowly exhale, relaxing the muscles. Try that two or three times. You'll notice that as you exhale, your whole body will relax and loosen up.

The final stage of this muscle-relaxation procedure requires you to settle back in your chair and get as comfortable as you can. Close your eyes and let all of your muscles become loose, limp, and completely relaxed. Let yourself go! Review each of these muscle groups in your mind and relax them as much as you can:

1. Hands and arms
2. Neck
3. Jaws, face, forehead
4. Shoulders and back
5. Stomach
6. Legs
7. Chest

Do not tense and tighten these muscles again. Concentrate solely on relaxing them. Keep your mind blank. Think only of your muscles. If any one muscle group is not as relaxed as the others, give that group more attention. After all your muscles are as relaxed as you can get them, take them one step further. Really give it all you've got. Let yourself go as you've never done before. When you're really relaxed you'll feel like a soggy noodle. If you're dieting, you'd better forget about the noodle and think about being a wet dishrag. Your whole body should feel warm and heavy. Enjoy the relaxation for about ten minutes and then proceed to Phase 2.

Don't be alarmed if you can't get *completely* relaxed. After all, this is the first time. With practice you'll soon be so proficient you'll become totally relaxed within five minutes or less. I want you to become so skilled at relaxation you'll become *addicted* to it forever. Then you'll never need your old addiction again. In fact, the pleasure you once derived from smoking, eating, or drinking will seem negligible compared to your newly discovered ability to relax.

PHASE 2: INTERNAL RELAXATION

Now that your muscles are relaxed, let's relax your internal organs. Take a deep breath, just as you did a moment ago. Exhale very slowly. Now breathe slowly and steadily. Just breathe naturally. Be aware of the entire sequence of your breathing process. Concentrate on inhaling and exhaling. Block everything else out of your mind. Listen to yourself breathe. *Feel* yourself breathe. Pay attention to the experience of breathing and the sensations in your chest, throat, mouth, and nose as you inhale and exhale. *Total concentration is essential.* Think only about breathing, and nothing else. After a few minutes make a conscious attempt to slow your breathing. Try to take shallow rather than deep breaths. Keep your body *completely* relaxed and limp as you do this. Take slow, shallow breaths until your breathing is relaxed and comfortable. Don't slow your breathing too much so that you're gasping for breath or your breathing is labored. Slow it down until it feels natural for you.

Concentrating on breathing may be a new experience for you. After all, how many of us go around thinking about how we breathe? You may have to become accustomed to this procedure before you feel comfortable with it. In fact, some people actually begin to feel a little anxious when they're doing this. One patient of mine became upset because she thought she might actually make herself stop breathing altogether. I assured her that that would *not* happen. Without realizing it, she really became frightened over the unexpected control she had over the internal functions of her body. Once she became used to this newly developed self-control her anxiety was replaced by a feeling bordering on ecstasy. The pleasure of being able to control your body completely can be extremely enjoyable.

To enhance this internal control process, say each of the following sentences to yourself:

> My breathing is slowing down.
> My heart rate is slowing down.
> I am feeling more and more relaxed.
> I have complete control over my body.

Repeat each sentence four or five times, saying it slowly and deliberately. Do not allow any other thoughts to interfere with your concentration. Nothing else is important right now. Don't think about what you have to do tomorrow or what happened this morning. Actively block these thoughts. Think of this relaxation procedure as a flight from the real world, as a 20- to 30-minute mental vacation from your life. You must focus on relaxation all the energies you usually expend on day-to-day mental and physical activities. You must "turn inward" and shut out the world about you. The sound of the dog barking or the kids arguing doesn't help; that's why it's important to choose a time for relaxation during which you'll have minimal distractions.

As you become adept at total relaxation you will automatically shut out distractions. Your senses simply will not respond to external stimuli while you're concentrating on relaxation. This may seem strange or perhaps impossible, but such experiences occur all the time. Total concentration on reading material can cause amnesia for other sensory inputs. The same thing happens during a strenuous athletic event or during a crisis. A professional football player may be so intensely involved in a game that he might not even feel pain from injuries. Several cases have occurred in which someone involved in an accident will save the lives of several other victims without realizing that he himself is seriously injured. Intense concentration can block feelings of pain and fear.

PHASE 3: MENTAL RELAXATION

Now that your body is relaxed—inside and out—let's relax your mind. This may be the *most* difficult form of relaxation for you, especially if you had trouble concentrating during Phases 1 and 2. Total concentration, the ability to block out all extraneous stimuli, is an ability not everyone possesses. Actually, you must learn to block external stimuli, such as television, the children, or the dog, as I have discussed above. However, even when it's completely quiet, when nobody is around to disturb you, *internal* stimuli may serve as distractions. That's right. Your own thoughts that are not related to the relaxation procedure may intrude. In the middle of your muscle-relaxing exercises you may find yourself thinking, "I'd better hurry up—I've got a lot to do today." *Stop* right there! *Relaxation* must be considered one of the most important aspects of your life. I'm afraid some of your old attitudes toward the productive use of time may hinder your progress in using this procedure. You *must* accept these facts:

It's important to relax and do absolutely nothing for 20 minutes each day.
Relaxation is probably *the* most important activity of your day.

Why do I say that it's okay to relax each day? Why is it necessary for you to give yourself permission to relax? Well, it's because you may be, as many people are, a goal-oriented, time-oriented, achievement-oriented individual. This can be true of you whether you're a clerk, secretary, vice-president, housewife, or laborer. Certainly there is nothing wrong with achievement. In fact, personal accomplishment through hard work is to be commended. But you don't have to be on the go every minute. In fact if one of your goals is a long, healthy life, then the regular practice of relaxation is one way to accomplish that goal. By relaxing for 20 minutes you're preventing yourself from smoking, eating, or drinking during that time.

In addition to working on changing your attitudes about relaxation, you will also have to condition yourself to feel comfortable when relaxing. This is a relatively simple process. Begin by shortening your relaxation sessions to about 5 minutes each. As soon as your mind starts wandering, *immediately* stop relaxing and call it quits. Later on that day, or the next day, try it again. Try to extend your periods of relaxation and concentration each day until you can block out the world for 20 minutes. If, at the beginning, 5 minutes is too long, then shorten the time to 2 minutes or even one minute. One full minute of deep relaxation is better than 10 minutes during which you're only partially relaxed.

Now, once you are *physically* relaxed, you can begin to train your mind to relax by mentally focusing on a specific word, picture, or symbol. Hypnotists often use this procedure to induce a hypnotic state. Those of you who have tried transcendental meditation have your own special mantra that you say to yourself. Any word or mental picture will do. I usually ask patients to think about the words "Relax" or "Calm." Close your eyes for a minute and get your mind totally blank. Now imagine the word "Relax" written in your mind. Try to see the word clearly and distinctly. As you look at the word, say "Relax" to yourself very slowly and clearly as if you were instructing yourself, *commanding* yourself to relax. Say the word over and over again. Say it slowly and softly. Say "Relax . . . Re-lax . . . Re-la-x . . . Re—la—x." Good! Each time you say the word, imagine that you're feeling more and more relaxed.

Thinking of a word such as this serves three purposes. First, it serves as a self-instruction, which puts *you* in charge of the relaxation process. You're taking an *active* part in relaxing yourself. Second, the word "Relax" serves as a *cue*, a trigger for a feeling of relaxation. The more you use this same word, the more it will become associated with a relaxed feeling. Just as certain cues trigger off your habit, the word "Relax" will begin to trigger off a relaxed feeling. You are conditioning yourself. Then when you need to relax quickly—to avoid a cigarette, for example—thinking of the word "Relax" will start off the sequence of bodily events necessary to relax you. If this sounds a bit as if you've been brainwashed, it's because you have been. Only, as I mentioned even at the beginning of this book, *you* are brainwashing yourself; and that's exactly what I'm teaching you to do. The third purpose of the word "Relax" is that it serves to focus your attention on the task at hand and away from distractions. You may find that when you try to keep your mind completely "blank," ideas, words, and pictures pop into your head. Thinking of nothing is difficult. By thinking of and concentrating on *something,* such as a word, you are keeping yourself from thinking of anything else. In addition to words, thoughts of pleasant situations can enhance your feelings of mental relaxation. Let me give you an example. I will describe a scene and I want you to think about it in great detail. Imagine that the situation is actually happening to you. Do *not* visualize it as if you were watching a movie, but rather as if you were experiencing the events right now. For example, if I were to tell you that you're standing in front of a tree, visualize the tree, its leaves, the ground around it, and the surrounding terrain. Use your mind's eye as a camera. Don't picture yourself looking at a tree. This distinction is important in terms of the degree of relaxation you'll experience. Also, make sure you use all your senses when imagining the scene. If you were imagining running along the beach, you should not only see the sand, ocean, and sky but also hear the waves, smell the salt air, and even feel the sand under your feet. Here's a scene that I often ask people to imagine while relaxing.

> You are walking through the woods on a very pleasant, sunny day. You're all alone, feeling relaxed, calm, and totally peaceful. Look all around you. Look up at the trees above you. Notice how full and green the branches are. Take a deep breath and smell the fresh country air. Stop for a moment and listen. Birds are singing off in the distance. Their sounds are cheerful.
>
> As you walk farther on, you notice, over to your right, a narrow babbling brook running through the woods. It's a small, shallow stream and you can hear the water over the stony bottom. Walk over to the stream and kneel down beside it. Put one hand in the water and feel its coolness. The water feels very cool and refreshing. The coolness

has a relaxing effect on you and you feel very calm. Now reach down into the water and pick up one of the small, smooth stones from the bottom. Take it firmly in your hand and stand up. The stone is very cool, very smooth and rounded. Rub the stone between your hands. Feel its texture. Now throw the stone back into the stream. Notice the splash it makes as it enters the water. Concentrate on the spot where it went into the water. Try to lose yourself mentally in the swirling stream of water. Let yourself relax and enjoy the surroundings.

Now start walking again. As you walk, try to feel the relaxation in your body. With each step you take you're becoming more and more relaxed.

Stop once again and look at all the fallen leaves on the ground. Pick up one of the leaves, one of the larger ones, and hold it in your hand. Rub it between your thumb and fingers. Feel the texture. Look at the leaf closely. Notice the colors. Bring it up to your nose and smell it. Take a deep breath. Now let the leaf drop from your hand. Continue walking slowly along. Feel the relaxation in your body, the heavy, warm feelings in your muscles.

Just in front of you the woods comes to an end. You see a clearing ahead. As you get closer to it you notice that you're standing at the edge of a huge meadow. The meadow has grassy hills as far as the eye can see. Green grassy hills. Throughout the meadow are beautiful wild flowers of every color and description. It's a gorgeous sight. As you walk into the meadow you notice the bright blue sky. The sun is very bright and warm and you can feel its warmth on your skin. It warms your whole body and relaxes you even more. You feel a slight warm breeze on your cheek. It's very gentle, very relaxing.

You walk toward a huge oak tree in the middle of the meadow. You walk slowly and steadily. When you get there, you lie down under the tree. As you lie down you're amazed to find that the ground is very, very soft. It doesn't feel as if you're lying on the ground at all. You

feel as if you are suspended, as if you're floating. As you
look up through the branches of the tree you notice again
how blue the sky is. There are just a few white fluffy
clouds drifting by. You get the feeling that you're floating
right along with those clouds. As you lie there looking
at the sky you feel more relaxed than you've ever felt
before. Your muscles are warm and relaxed. You feel
calm and peaceful, without a care in the world.

Most people don't want to come back to reality after this
mental journey. With practice you'll be able to go in and out
of these imaginings quickly and easily. Remember, concentrate
on experiencing the sequence of events clearly and vividly.
Make use of all your senses and emotions. As you imagine this
situation, keep your muscles relaxed and your breathing
slowed.

Give some thought to other scenes that might be pleasant
and relaxing for you. How about sailing, walking on the beach
at sunset, horseback riding, skiing, floating on a raft in the
middle of a lake? Choose a *relaxing* scene, not an exciting or
stimulating one. Also, be *alone* in the situation. If you're with
someone else, that person's presence can evoke thoughts and
feelings that might distract you.

CONTROLLING CRAVINGS THROUGH RELAXATION

As I mentioned previously, the phenomenon of craving has
both cognitive and physical characteristics. When you crave a
cigarette, a Scotch, or a candy bar, your mind *and* your body
react. You battle with yourself about the merits of continued
habit control versus the immediate pleasure that one small
overindulgence would bring. Your muscles tense, your heart
rate speeds up, and you feel momentarily out of control of the
situation. Food, cigarettes, or alcohol serve to reduce these un-

pleasant sensations almost immediately. Relaxation, however, can do the same thing. It can actually eliminate the craving by partially satisfying it.

To demonstrate the amount of control you have over cravings, try to use your imagination to visualize a hypothetical situation. The scene I'll describe is for dieters, so merely substitute a cigarette or alcohol if you're a smoker or drinker.

> You are at home alone, feeling very bored and restless. You don't expect anybody else to come home for several hours. Imagine yourself walking into the kitchen. You open the refrigerator and take out one of your very favorite foods. You place it on the kitchen table and sit down in front of it. Look at the food closely. Think about how good it would taste. Smell it, look at it.

As you conjure up this image, concentrate on your feelings. What is happening in your muscles, your stomach, your mouth? Do you have an "empty" feeling in your stomach as you think about the food? Are you getting tense? Do you feel even a little bit uneasy? If your imagination is vivid enough, you'll be able to develop an intense craving by using this mental exercise.

Once you are aware of your feelings, examine them closely. A key to successful habit control lies in being able to recognize exactly how cravings affect you. You must be able to differentiate between cravings and feelings of general tension, depression, or boredom.

Now that a craving is present, you can eliminate it by going through the relaxation procedure. Go through each phase, relaxing your muscles, internal organs, and mind. Pay particular attention to those parts of your body in which you are experiencing your craving the most. For example, if an "empty" feeling is associated with your cravings for food, concentrate on relaxing your stomach. Be sure to tighten and then relax your stomach muscles several times. Think about the feelings in your stomach. Repeat such phrases as:

My stomach is calm and relaxed.
My stomach is full and comfortable.
I feel very content and satisfied.
My stomach muscles are loose and relaxed.

Cravings for cigarettes and alcohol are not usually localized in one area of the body. Rather, these cravings are experienced as general, over-all uneasiness and tension. Some smokers, however, report that during cravings for a cigarette the mouth, nose, throat, and lungs feel "different." This is usually a vague, uncomfortable feeling that is difficult to describe, but the sensation is there nevertheless. Drinkers occasionally report sensations of thirst when they crave alcohol. The important thing is to determine what *your* craving is and how it makes *you* feel.

If smoking is your problem, concentrate on total muscular relaxation. Then take several deep breaths, exhaling each very slowly. Try to develop a very easy, relaxed style of breathing. Also focus your attention on your throat and neck muscles. Tense and relax them several times, telling yourself repeatedly:

My throat is totally relaxed.
My breathing is slowing down.
My throat and neck muscles are loose and limp.

Repeat this craving-relaxation sequence about three times a week for at least a month. Also use the relaxation procedure to cope with day-to-day cravings that occur spontaneously. You can use a modified version of the procedure to initiate rapid control when you don't have time to run through the 20-

minute sequence. Suppose a craving hits when you're driving to work, visiting a friend, or attending a meeting? Simply becoming more aware of your physical and mental state at that time may be sufficient to control the urge. Let's suppose you're driving past a familiar tavern on your way home. You start thinking about having a few drinks. You can almost taste them. Your cravings are very strong. *Don't panic.* Immediately take a quick personal inventory by asking yourself the following questions:

1. Are my muscles tight and tense?
2. Have my breathing and heart rates increased?
3. What specific words, pictures, or ideas are in my mind?
4. Do my mouth and throat feel dry?
5. Are my mouth and throat muscles tense?

Now, on the basis of your answers to this self-evaluation, relax those parts of your body that need relaxing the most. Let your muscles loosen up. Distract your mind by visualizing a relaxing scene. Concentrate on the word "Relax." Very soon, sometimes in less than a minute, you'll discover that you have eliminated your craving completely. The more practice you have at disposing of cravings through relaxation, the better you'll become at it.

Recreation and Exercise

In addition to relaxation, recreational activities and exercise are excellent alternatives to substance abuse. Now, I'm not necessarily talking about *strenuous* sports or exercises, but enjoyable ones. You must choose these types of alternatives carefully so that they don't become a chore for you. Remember, you are using alternatives as a substitute for eating, smoking, or drinking. They *must* be at least minimally pleasurable for you.

When changing your habits and developing a more active life style in the process, you must avoid overdoing it. Starting a new habit that is good for you is almost as difficult as stopping one that's bad. How many times have you started a daily jogging régime and failed to continue it? The first two mornings are probably great. You're up at 7:00 A.M. running around the neighborhood, feeling healthy and smug. You probably wonder why you quit jogging the last time you took it up. Well, after the second morning your muscles are sore all over, your legs ache, and you find you're in a lot worse physical condition than you thought. On the third morning you're a bit sleepy after the party the night before. You really don't feel like getting out of bed, much less jogging, but you force yourself. Once you get going you feel better and you're proud of yourself for not staying in bed. You stick to your routine on the fourth and fifth days although your initial enthusiasm is wearing off. Jogging by yourself is *so* boring for you. On the sixth day it's raining, so you decide to skip your morning jog and do it that evening. Somehow you never get the chance, because it's "one of those days." The seventh day is cold and overcast and you feel very sleepy and sluggish. You decide to skip it again. You jog the next morning, but the two-day layoff has made you tire easily. The jogging seems especially hard on you this morning. You end up jogging only half your usual distance and wondering whether all this exercise is really worth it. Then, before you know it, you're not jogging anymore. Well, don't feel too bad. In fact, your behavior is very typical. Old habits, such as staying in bed to a reasonable hour in the morning, are very difficult to break.

WHERE TO BEGIN

The first step in planning recreational alternatives to over-consumption is to remember some basic rules of thumb:

1. Develop a variety of activities rather than one or two.
2. Make certain your activities are *enjoyable* ones.
3. Include some activities that can be done alone and some with others.
4. *Begin gradually* to acclimatize yourself to your new activities.
5. *Never* plan an activity that is incompatible with your present life style.

Before you do anything else, survey the possible alternatives available to you. Develop a list of activities that you think you might enjoy. When compiling your list, don't limit yourself to the few recreational activities that you occasionally engage in. Your goal should be to expand your horizons. Do a little brainstorming and use your imagination. When considering possibilities, *do not* rule out an activity, such as tennis, just because you're not skilled at it. *Do not* rule out something even if you have *no* training or skill in that activity. When compiling your list consider these sources:

1. Activities in which you were once active but no longer participate
2. Activities that you've always wanted to participate in, but because of procrastination or lack of skill, have never tried
3. Activities that your friends or family participate in but you don't
4. Activities that you engage in only occasionally

On this basis you should be able to get up a list of at least fifteen to twenty recreational and exercise activities. Let's suppose that your list looks something like this:

Horseback riding
Tennis
Walking
Jogging
Bicycling
Handball
Golf
Calisthenics
Woodworking
Furniture refinishing
Solving crossword puzzles
Chess
Coin collecting
Painting
Sculpturing
Writing poetry and short stories

Notice that this list includes a wide range of sports, hobbies, exercises, and general recreational activities. While some include planning, most are readily available and would be continuously accessible to you.

For the next couple of months you should sample the majority of activities on your list. Don't make any commitments about getting involved in any of them. Just sample each one to see how enjoyable it might be. Do *not* make up your mind ahead of time that you're not going to like something or that you won't be proficient at something. Give each activity an equal chance even if you've tried it before. And don't think you have to be skilled at something to enjoy it. You may be a lousy tennis player and still enjoy tennis immensely.

Make certain you participate in each activity at least once even if you've never done it before. Take a couple of golf lessons, go horseback riding, get someone to teach you to play chess, buy an old piece of junk furniture and fix it up, paint a picture, write a poem. If you don't like an activity at first, give it a chance. Try it a time or two more. If you still don't like it, then cross it off your list.

Once you narrow your list down, start to participate in these activities regularly. Plan them for times when you are most likely to be smoking, eating, or drinking. Have your paints, writing tablet, or woodworking tools readily available to help distract you when cravings occur.

WALKING—THE BEST ACTIVITY

I must admit that I'm a little biased when it comes to recreational activities. My own preference, above all others, is for walking. This is not to say that you don't need a variety of alternatives. It's just that walking is enjoyable to just about everybody and available to almost everyone. No matter what shape you're in, you can walk. Walking can also get you in shape for other, more strenuous activities, such as jogging or handball. By going for a long walk when you feel like having a cigarette, you're removing yourself from the source of temptation *and* providing yourself with a pleasant activity. Walking will eliminate your tension and craving. Many people find walking and light jogging incompatible with substance use. That is, immediately after these activities, eating, smoking, or drinking is simply not enjoyable to them.

You can make walking a challenge by exploring different neighborhoods, parks, or interesting downtown areas of your city. My father, who is a retired business executive, stays active by meeting with a friend twice a week to walk. They plan these outings very carefully (using a city map), driving to different locations in the community to vary their walking surroundings. It's amazing how many new and interesting locations you can discover this way.

You can also make walking a challenge by keeping track of the number of miles you walk each day. You can monitor these miles with the use of a pedometer, a small device you wear at your waist which records mileage based on the number of steps you take. Pedometers can be purchased at any local sporting goods store. For those who want to be classy, Tiffany's carries a sterling silver model that is quite elegant.

Whatever activity you choose, practice it routinely so that it becomes as important in your life as your old habit once was.

CHAPTER SIX

You May Be Your Own Worst Enemy

If I were to ask why you just lit up a cigarette after going two days without one, you might say, "Because I had an overwhelming desire to smoke and couldn't resist." Actually, you might have talked yourself into it, and failed to realize what happened because you weren't listening to your thoughts. Certainly you sometimes reach for a cigarette or a potato chip with little or no thought of what you're doing. The classic example of this is the smoker who lights up a cigarette only to find that he still has another, half smoked, lying in the ashtray. Such occurences, however, are infrequent. Most of your behavior follows a series of thoughts related to your decision to light up, eat, or drink. You simply have not trained yourself to recognize these thoughts and their powerful influence on you. Also, like most people, you are more than ready to attribute your "loss of control" to some irresistible force within you rather than to your own conscious decision-making process. We're all experts at letting ourselves off the hook.

Exactly what are these irresistible forces? These urges? These cravings? Partly they are a series of thoughts that influence your decision to smoke, eat, or drink. An urge can begin with a physiological craving, as the result of physical

137

addiction. It may take the form of nervousness, irritability, or hunger pangs. Urges, however, do not directly result in putting something into your mouth. Rather, they influence *thoughts* about your habit. These thoughts take you one step closer to overconsumption. For example, your "growling" stomach may bring to mind the last time you ate in your favorite Italian restaurant. You can picture the food in front of you. You can almost smell and taste it. These visual and gustatory thoughts trigger off verbal thoughts. You think to yourself, "I'll die if I don't have just one piece of pizza. One little piece won't hurt me. I'll eat less food for dinner to make up for it." Guess what? You just talked yourself into a family-sized pepperoni pizza, two beers, and a devastating feeling of guilt.

You *can* learn to control urges and thoughts. It *is* possible; you're just not used to doing it. Remember, no one ever went crazy from a "nicotine fit" or fainted from the lack of a piece of cake!

Let's examine basic thought processes that precede your loss of control, and what you can do to change them.

Thoughts About Food, Cigarettes, or Alcohol

Most overconsumption is the direct result of your active imagination. A mental image of a cigarette may pop into your mind after breakfast, a time when you used to enjoy smoking with your morning coffee. You might see a pack of cigarettes clearly in your mind. You might vicariously experience the pleasure of smoking a cigarette in your imagination.

These mental images are often triggered by external sources —certain times of the day or situations that have in the past been associated with your habit. You may find that you think most about having a drink during the "cocktail hour," just before your evening meal. Even conversation can trigger urges. John may overhear his coworkers discussing the seven-course gourmet meal they had at a dinner party the previous evening. Sarah may hear several friends expressing pleasure and relief when they are finally able to light cigarettes at the intermission of a lengthy play. Neither John nor Sarah may have been thinking of food or cigarettes until faced with these situations. Now each may find that, at least for several minutes or hours, the object of their addictions becomes an obsession. Both John and Sarah must develop a plan of action to counteract these images. This plan must be well rehearsed before the need arises for its use.

THE "ULTIMATE CONSEQUENCES" TECHNIQUE

One effective method of thought control involves the ultimate consequences of your behavior. Specifically, I'm referring to the positive effects of successful and permanent habit control (for example, clothes will fit better if I lose weight) and the negative effects of continued overconsumption (for example, lung cancer or heart attack). Unfortunately, you are much more influenced by short-term consequences of your behavior than long-term ones. Who ever thinks of dying from lung cancer in twenty years while enjoying the first satisfying puff of a cigarette? In addition, the immediate effects of consumption are positive and usually override considerations of any long-term negative effects. You probably don't give much thought to ultimate behavioral consequences until *after* you have smoked, eaten, or drunk. Then—only after you've consumed the substance—you begin thinking about the effects it has on you. But it's too late! All those thoughts do for you then is give you a massive case of frustration and guilt. In turn, guilt feelings trigger off more consumption. You think,

"Why did I smoke that cigarette? Dr. Long told me I had to quit, or else. What's the use. I'm so upset now I'll just have to wait until Monday to quit."

In order to use ultimate consequences beneficially, you must examine them closely. Let's begin with the eventual negative effects of your habit. Remember, I'm talking about long-term effects. For example, suppose you continue to drink heavily for the rest of your life. In fact, imagine that each year of your life you increase your consumption until you're drinking large amounts of alcohol every day. If you are a smoker, imagine that you smoke more each year, perhaps consuming up to five or six packs of cigarettes each day. For you dieters, imagine that you gain ten pounds each year for the next five years. Now think of all the possible effects of this continued overconsumption on your physical health, psychological well-being, and/or personal appearance. Write the five worst consequences on one side of a small index card. Make sure they are very specific and meaningful to you. Sample lists of three individuals, each with a different habit problem, are presented below.

Don's Smoking List—Negative Consequences
1. Lung cancer
2. Heart attack
3. Stained teeth and fingers
4. Son's adoption of smoking habit when he is older
5. Worsening of chronic cough

Virginia's Overeating List—Negative Consequences
1. High blood pressure
2. Heart attack

3. Physical unattractiveness
4. Depression
5. Increased self-consciousness

Paul's Drinking List—Negative Consequences
1. Cirrhosis of the liver
2. Cancer of the esophagus
3. Marital problems
4. Financial expense
5. Deterioration of job performance

Now turn your index card over and write five *positive* consequences of successful habit control. Consider what would happen if you never again had to worry about controlling your habit. Imagine that you have quit smoking completely and will never smoke again for the rest of your life. Or think about losing all your excess fat and maintaining an ideal weight forever. Let your imagination wander and consider every possible positive influence that this permanent change would have on your life. Let's examine the positive consequences listed by Don, Virginia, and Paul.

Don's Smoking List—Positive Consequences
1. Longer life
2. Better taste to food
3. Feeling of personal accomplishment
4. Improved stamina in physical activities
5. Better quality of physical health with age

Virginia's Overeating List—Positive Consequences
1. Longer life
2. Improved health

3. Increased participation in recreational activities
4. Greater social activity
5. Availability of stylish clothes in smaller sizes

Paul's Drinking List—Positive Consequences
1. Improved health
2. Feeling of personal accomplishment
3. Better concentration
4. Improved family relations
5. Improved sexual performance

Now make a duplicate card of your lists. Keep one card with you at all times. Keep the other card in a prominent place at home or at work. Tape it to the refrigerator door, prop it up on your desk, put it by the telephone, or tape it to your liquor cabinet. Every time you have a mental image of food, cigarettes, or alcohol, take out your list and read over each item. Consider each one carefully. Don't rush through the list. You are going to use these ultimate consequences to counteract powerful thoughts and urges. To do this successfully you must make an emotional impact on yourself. You can't fight off a strong urge to overeat with a fleeting thought of something that may not happen to you for five years.

As an illustration of the specifics of this technique, let's consider how Don might use his "ultimate consequences" lists to keep from smoking. Don is a forty-year-old attorney who is happily married, with two teenage children. In his youth he was very active and athletic and proud of his physical stamina. He played baseball in college, married a childhood sweetheart, and studied law at the University of Virginia. His winning personality and high scholastic standing landed him a position with a well-established law firm in New York City. Being energetic, he worked hard and became a partner. Even though he's finally made it, Don can't help feeling a little down in the dumps lately. He doesn't seem as motivated as he once was. He has little vitality and becomes short of breath with the least amount of exertion. Don decides to have a complete medical examination—something he has avoided for years. His physician discovers a significant reduction in lung capacity and warns Don about the possibility of emphysema. Don is shocked by this news. He has been warned before about the possible health risks of his heavy smoking. His three-pack-a-day habit is finally catching up with him. Don is determined to quit smoking in order to improve and prolong the quality of his life. In addition to the health risk, it bothers him that a small amount of tobacco wrapped in thin white paper can have so much control over him.

In order to gain control over urges to smoke, Don employs the "ultimate consequences" lists described above. He keeps one index card in his shirt pocket and one propped up against the ashtray on his desk at work. One day at the office Don has a strong craving to smoke. He begins thinking about how good a cigarette would taste. He's so obsessed with this thought that he can't concentrate on the letters he is dictating. Don immediately picks up the index card and reads the first negative consequence on his list: "Lung cancer." Don realizes that he must really imagine himself experiencing this eventual effect of smoking for it to counteract his cravings. He closes his eyes and imagines himself lying in a hospital bed, with a physician and nurse in attendance. The doctor is telling him that he has cancer of the lung and that the cancer is spreading all over his body. He has six months to live, perhaps a year at the most. Don can see his wife standing by his bedside crying. Don feels very upset, depressed, and helpless as he lies there.

Don then goes to the next consequence: "Heart attack." He imagines the pain and agony of having a heart attack and being rushed to the hospital. Thus he works his way through the list, vividly imagining each consequence as if it were happening right then. He imagines his son beginning to smoke, in order to be like his dad. He even thinks about the eventual detrimental health effects smoking will have on his son. He imagines his son having a heart attack because of excessive smoking.

Next Don turns the index card over and reads each positive consequence. As he reads Item 4 he pictures himself playing two sets of tennis without getting out of breath. He breathes in deeply and is proud of his new stamina. For Item 5 he imagines himself at seventy years of age. His physician is telling him that he's in great shape.

By the time Don has imagined each negative and positive item on his list, thoughts of smoking are gone. He has a stronger resolve to keep from smoking. He replaces his index card on the desk and is ready to use it again when he needs it.

In Don's case, health and physical stamina were important consequences for him. For another person other factors, such as personal appearance, might be as meaningful as or more meaningful than long-term health considerations. This is often true for dieters. A dieter might have as Item 1 on her list "Being physically unattractive." Here she should imagine herself naked and thirty pounds heavier than her present weight. As she stands in front of a mirror she sees the rolls of fat, the bulges. She experiences feelings of disgust and embarrassment. On the positive side, being able to buy and wear attractive clothes is important to dieters. Overweight individuals are well aware that most stores have a very limited selection of clothing in the larger sizes. Perhaps two black dresses that would have been in style ten years ago! If this item is on your list, imagine yourself in an expensive clothing store. Without asking your size the saleswoman takes you over to the size 10 dresses. You feel exhilarated. Imagine trying on several stylish outfits. Imagine yourself in a slinky white dress that hugs your slender body. You can see yourself clearly in the mirror; you can feel the excitement.

The key to success with this procedure is total concentration and total sensory experience. You must see, hear, and *feel* what you are imagining. Make believe the consequence is occurring *right now*—not ultimately, but *now*. Always begin with the negative consequences and conclude with the positive ones. Ending on a positive note will put you in a better frame of mind. After all, Personal Habit Control consists of positive steps; learning positive behavior skills to change habits. Your ultimate goal is to replace negative habits with more positive ones. Similarly, your new *thinking* habits should emphasize positive motivational aspects more than negative ones. In fact, as I'll discuss later in this chapter, one of your bad habits might be too much negative thinking.

If you practice this technique consistently, thoughts of ultimate consequences will pop into your head automatically whenever you are tempted to overindulge. You'll no longer need to refer to your written lists. In a sense, you are emotionally conditioning your thought patterns through constant repetition of this cognitive routine.

During the early stages of your habit-change program it's a good idea to keep these consequences in mind whether or not you're being tempted. During the first two weeks you should read through your lists once a day regardless of your urges. If you find that one or two consequences lose their impact because of constant repetition, have some alternate consequences available.

When you use the "ultimate consequences" technique

List only consequences that are personally meaningful to you.

Keep your list with you at all times.

Visualize each consequence as *vividly* and *emotionally* as possible.

Always think of your positive consequences last.

COGNITIVE CONDITIONING

A second technique to control urges is called *cognitive conditioning* or *covert sensitization*. In this procedure you condition your thoughts by consciously associating food, cigarettes, or alcohol with very unpleasant and repulsive thoughts. The rationale behind this technique is that thoughts can be modified in much the same way that behavior is modified. When a child is burned by touching a hot stove, his stove-touching behavior will be modified. Because of this negative association he is less likely to touch the stove again.

Your behavior is conditioned in this way all the time. Generally, you are more likely to behave in ways that lead to or are associated with pleasurable occurrences and less likely to do things that are associated with negative occurrences. Of course, human behavior is far from being that simple, but as a rule many of your habitual behaviors are learned in this manner. Perhaps you have had a past experience in which a certain food has developed negative associations. Perhaps your mother made you eat liver because it was "good for you," even though you had to force it down. Now, as an adult, the

mere sight of liver is enough to make you sick. That's a natural example of what is sometimes referred to as *aversion
conditioning*.

Your thoughts follow the same conditioning principles.
Only you've been conditioning yourself in the wrong direction.
You've been associating thoughts of alcohol with the pleasurable sensations derived from drinking. First you think about
a beer, then you drink one, then you experience pleasure.
After repeated associations of the thought, behavior, and
positive consequence, the thought itself brings about the same
pleasurable sensation (or at least the expectations of the
sensation) as the behavior does. Thoughts of alcoholic beverages will then occur more frequently.

Your habit-control goal is to repeatedly associate thoughts
about food, cigarettes, or alcohol with a very negative experience. Every time you see a cigarette or think about one,
conjure up a negative thought. In a sense, punish yourself in
your mind for having these thoughts. By doing this you will
reduce the number of urges you have and thus make habit
control an easier task. If you do this often enough you may
find that you lose much of your desire for and interest in food,
cigarettes, or alcohol.

Let's assume that you are doing well controlling your
smoking, with the exception of periodic cravings for a cigarette. Whenever you see somebody smoking a cigarette, it
drives you crazy. In this case you should schedule a time every
day when you cognitively condition yourself. You are going
to break the association between cigarettes and pleasurable
taste. First, imagine yourself in a familiar situation in which
cigarettes are available. Perhaps you are at a friend's home
and she is smoking. Further, imagine in detail and with great
emotionality, the following sequence of events:

You're sitting with your friend, looking at her intently as she takes a puff of her cigarette and inhales deeply. An open pack of cigarettes is lying on the coffee table in front of you. As you smell the smoke from her cigarette you get a tremendous urge to have just one drag. She offers you a cigarette and you accept. As you light up, the smoke begins to burn your mouth and throat. You feel light-headed and dizzy. You're weak all over. You feel as if you are going to faint. You see spots in front of your eyes and your vision is blurred. You're very, very dizzy. As you take another drag you begin to cough and choke. The smoke makes your sinuses drain into your throat. Your burning throat is filled with mucus. Clots of phlegm are caught in your throat. You're gagging and trying to swallow the phlegm. You begin coughing. It's a hacking cough that brings the phlegm into your mouth. You are getting sick to your stomach. You try to swallow the mucus and its gets stuck in your throat again. Now you're really gagging. Smoke is all around you. Phlegm is sliding up and down your throat. You're dizzy and your eyes and mouth increasingly feel as if they are on fire. You gag and choke and gasp for a breath. As you take one more drag and inhale, a crushing pain hits your chest. The choking doesn't let up. You feel as if a thousand-pound weight is on your chest. Suddenly you feel another sharp, agonizing pain in the center of your chest. The pain is unbearable. You're fighting for breath but you can barely breathe at all. You begin to panic. You're gasping faster and faster. You can't stand it much longer.

After imagining this situation, rest for a minute or two, and then go over it again four or five more times. Go through this procedure several times, especially during the first two or three weeks of your habit-control program. Change the scene from time to time, picturing and trying to enter into different unpleasant experiences. Don't be concerned about how realistic or unrealistic the situation is. The more severe and drastic the experience is, the more likely it is to influence you. People often say to me, "But this will never happen to me." It doesn't matter. It only matters that you vividly experience these sensations in your mind in association with thoughts of smoking. Remember to let yourself really experience these events in your imagination. Try to really feel yourself choking and the panic when you're gasping for breath.

Even though all this may sound a bit ridiculous at first, many people find it very helpful. The more often you use this procedure, the more likely it is to reduce your urges. Repetition is the key.

It is also essential that you associate your thoughts with an experience that is truly horrendous for you. Try to personalize the experience. For example, a heavy drinker's greatest fear may be that someday he will be responsible for a tragic automobile accident while he is intoxicated. His cognitive conditioning session would include his drinking (perhaps while driving) and then causing an accident. He might clearly imagine the pain he feels, the blood all over his body, or his bloody leg, severed at the thigh!

A dieter might associate thoughts of nausea with foods that are particularly attractive to him.

> You walk into the drugstore thinking how delicious a candy bar will taste. Your craving for chocolate is irresistible. As you walk over to the candy counter, and as your craving gets stronger, you begin to feel a queasy sensation in the pit of your stomach. As you pick up the candy bar to look at it you feel a stronger wave of nausea coming over you. You pay for the candy bar and begin to walk out of the store. As you do, you start to feel very, very sick to your stomach. You can feel your stomach churning. There is an acid taste in your mouth and it is becoming difficult for you to swallow. You are now out

on the sidewalk unwrapping the candy. You think to yourself, "Maybe I'll feel better if I eat just one bite." You can see the chocolate very clearly. The chocolate smell is very strong. Rather than being pleasant, the smell is repulsive to you. Your stomach is churning even more. You begin to feel dizzy and light-headed. You feel your stomach heaving. You quickly take a bite of the candy bar. The taste is rotten and repugnant. You feel vomit coming up your throat and into your mouth. It burns your throat. You begin to vomit. Now the smell of vomit and chocolate are mixed together and you feel worse. You throw the candy away and vow never to eat candy again. In fact, any craving for chocolate has left you completely.

In addition to its use in thought control, covert conditioning can also assist you when you're directly confronted with temptation. What happens when you're faced with a cigarette, a second helping of your favorite casserole, or a Scotch on the rocks? In most instances, even though you are trying to resist, you're probably thinking about how good it looks or how good it would taste. You are ultrasensitive to the way that cigarette looks or the way the smoke streams out. When confronted in this way, immediately turn your thoughts to negative associations. Consider how dirty and messy the ashes are. Think about the cigarette as if it were poison. The smoke is toxic and even one puff may be deadly. If pie, rolls, or peanuts are your downfall, imagine something is wrong with them. As you look at these foods, use your creativity to think of ways to "spoil" them in your mind. Imagine that instead of pecans on that pie, the top is covered with large brown cockroaches. They are sitting very still, but as you look closely you can see one of them move slightly. Yes, I know, I'm asking you to train yourself to hallucinate. But hasn't your appetite for pecan pie decreased just a bit? Think that the rolls on your restaurant table are moldy. Thick green mold covers each one of them.

One of my dieting patients was concentrating on this technique at a cocktail party recently. The hostess, noticing her guest staring so intently at a bowl of peanuts, offered her some. My patient, who was still concentrating on her covert conditioning and only half aware of what was happening, replied, "No, thanks, there are worms crawling all over those peanuts!" Needless to say, the hostess was horrified and hurriedly checked all the rest of her food for worms.

Another dieter was a bit skeptical as I described this technique to her. She thought that imagining bugs all over her favorite food was quite silly. I insisted that she at least try the method a few times. She remained unconvinced. The day after our conversation she baked a chocolate cake for relatives and placed it in a cake tin while she did some shopping. Upon returning home she had a strong desire for one small piece of cake. To her amazement, when she took the top off the cake tin, her lovely chocolate cake was covered with ants! Live ants, that is, not imaginary ones. To this day she thinks I have some magical powers to make my covert conditioning scenes come true. I am happy to report that she lost all desire for chocolate cake after that and decided to use the technique after all.

I think you'll be amazed at how well covert conditioning works for you. Make a challenge of it. With each temptation, each craving, be determined to condition your thoughts and feelings through this process of association.

Self-Defeating Thoughts About Your Habit-Control Efforts

The first step in controlling self-defeating thought patterns is to become more aware of your thoughts. You should become particularly aware of thoughts occurring immediately prior to an episode of overconsumption. After you succumb to temptation, rather than feeling guilty and sorry for yourself, try a little self-analysis. Use the experience positively; learn from it. If you can pinpoint the sequence of negative thinking that resulted in consumption, you will be better able to prevent the same thing from happening again. It often helps to write down your thoughts.

Michael is a thirty-two-year-old assistant manager of a large department store. His wife, Cynthia, is thirty-one years old and a part-time college student. Cynthia put Michael through school working as a secretary and now wants to complete her own education. She has been under a lot of stress lately, trying to study and also care for their four-year-old daughter. Michael recently quit smoking and has been urging Cynthia to do the same. She argues that she is too tense to quit and will think about it later. Michael went two weeks without a cigarette, and then, one fateful Wednesday, he began smoking again. That evening Michael felt disgusted with himself. He had been doing so well. What had happened? He examined his thought patterns and his actions on that day. He had gotten up, come downstairs for breakfast, and had seen his wife drinking a cup of coffee and smoking a cigarette. From then until he finally lit a cigarette at the office his sequence of thoughts about smoking had gone as follows:

1. "I sure wish Cynthia would give up smoking. I've done it; why can't she?"
2. "She smokes about two packs a day. It's not fair that she can smoke and I have to quit."
3. "Why should I deprive myself of cigarettes? There

are so few pleasures in life. I should be enjoying my life as much as possible."

4. "I'm just weak-willed, anyway. Why should I continue to torture myself? I'll be smoking again sooner or later, so I might as well start now."

5. "My boss makes me so mad. I need a cigarette or I'll be a nervous wreck. Nobody could stop smoking with a job like mine."

Now that Michael is aware of his thoughts, he can begin to counteract them. In retrospect, Michael can now consider more positive arguments as replacements for the negative ones. For example, in place of statement No. 3 he could have argued, "Yes, but my life may be shorter if I continue to smoke. Besides, one of the pleasures in life is the knowledge that I can control my behavior." For No. 4 he could have said, "There is no such thing as being weak-willed. I can learn self-control if I really change my behavior and thought patterns."

Think about the last few episodes during which you talked yourself into filling your mouth. Write down specific thoughts that caused you trouble. Dieters usually discourage themselves most by thinking, "I stuck to my diet faithfully all week and didn't lose a pound. I'm just not losing fast enough." Smokers often tell themselves, "It's no use. I guess I'm just addicted. I'd rather be content as a smoker than always miserable and tense as a nonsmoker." As you can see, these are simply excuses or rationalizations that you use to make it more acceptable for you to overeat or smoke. It's actually amazing how skillful some people are at talking themselves into overindulgence.

Once you've listed at least four or five of your most typical excuses, write a positive thought to counteract each one. Ask yourself, "What would a panel of objective judges, interested in my welfare, say to me to help counteract my negative thinking?" Let's look at an example. The following is a list of four rationalizations used by a heavy drinker prior to having one too many. Next to each is a more positive statement to counteract the negative thought.

Negative Thought

1. "Everybody else is drinking a lot tonight. People will think I'm unsociable if I don't have a few more drinks."

2. "I need a few drinks to relax. I've had a rough day."

3. "I really blew it. I promised myself I wouldn't drink tonight and I had a beer. I might as well keep drinking

Positive Thought

1. "How much booze other people drink has nothing to do with my own drinking. If they think I'm unsociable just because I'm not drinking a lot, that's their problem, not mine."

2. "Two drinks is plenty to relax me. If I have any more I'll just get drunk and feel miserable tomorrow. Besides, I want to try out that new self-relaxation technique I learned last week."

3. "Just because I had one beer doesn't mean I have to continue drinking. I can stop right now. I'm not going to

Negative Thought	*Positive Thought*
and try again tomorrow."	let this small setback destroy everything I've accomplished all week."
4. "Ann and I are getting along better lately. I'd sure like to make love tonight. A few drinks will make sex more enjoyable for both of us."	4. "The reason Ann and I are getting along so well is because I'm not drinking as much. A few drinks will mess up everything. Besides, even though I feel more amorous when I'm drinking, I'm usually impotent after a few drinks."

Once you have written these positive thoughts next to the negative ones, learn them well. Study them. Memorize them. Then, whenever self-defeating thoughts enter your mind, counteract them immediately with your positive ones. Don't hesitate; do it as soon as you catch yourself making up excuses for yourself. Repeat the positive thought over and over again.

Now you are taking active steps toward developing and maintaining a positive attitude toward your habit-control efforts. Simply put, if you remain positive and avoid fooling yourself, you'll be successful. Because of the importance of a positive attitude, train yourself to think positive thoughts more often. Periodically, during the day, review your thoughts for the foregoing hour or two. Were you thinking negatively? Any such thoughts as "I'm not sure I can make it all day without a drink"? Were you making any such excuses as "I've been good all day. Maybe I should reward myself with just one cigarette"? If so, write down these thoughts immediately. What positive thoughts or arguments can you replace them with?

When you are first beginning to evaluate your thought processes, this hourly self-review process is a good idea. And it is helpful to provide yourself with an obvious reminder for you to review your thinking. For example, take a few minutes to review your thoughts each time you look at your watch or each time you have a cup of coffee. In this way you will remember and recognize negative thoughts more easily. This self-review method will also give you an indication of what times during the day you are most likely to let your thoughts get the best of you.

Self-Defeating Thoughts About Everyday Problems

Thoughts about everyday life problems very often precipitate episodes of overconsumption. This is especially true of the binge consumer, who controls himself for a period of time and then gorges himself with food, alcohol, or cigarettes when he is emotionally upset. In this situation, overconsumption is an attempt to find relief from boredom, depression, tension, or anger. Unfortunately, or perhaps fortunately, filling your mouth with any substance is not a cure for anger, depression, or tension. For example, the only *appropriate* stimulus for eating is hunger, not tension or boredom. While part of the solution to binge eating is learning real alternatives to problem solving and emotional release, another part is modifying irrational thought sequences that build up inappropriate strong emotions.

You must not allow your irrational thinking (and we're all guilty of this from time to time) to influence your efforts at habit control. Be more aware of everything you say to yourself. Question your thoughts. Counteract negative thoughts with techniques you have learned in this chapter. And remember, be on guard constantly, because, whether you like to admit it or not, *you may be (and probably are) your own worst enemy!*

Whenever you get a strong desire for a cigarette, a handful of peanuts, or a Bourbon on the rocks, ask yourself these questions:

> What am I saying to myself?
> Am I giving myself excuses?
> Am I thinking in a rational, logical manner?
> What negative images can I use to counteract this craving?
> What are the long-term consequences of my overconsumption?

Then say these two sentences to yourself *firmly* and *decisively:*

> My craving, even though it is a strong physical feeling, is caused in large part by my thoughts!
> I *can* and *will* control my thoughts!

CHAPTER SEVEN

─── Your Consummatory Style: Controlling Your Eating, Smoking, and Drinking

Consummatory style, or *how* you smoke, eat, and drink, is an important aspect of habit control. There is evidence to suggest that those who use substances to excess consume them very differently from moderate users. For example, let's examine the differences between heavy, problem drinkers and light-to-moderate drinkers. Certainly the former group drinks *more* alcohol than the latter group. There are also some interesting differences in the style of their drinking. Problem drinkers are more likely to drink straight drinks (that is, liquor with no mixer added), while moderate drinkers tend to drink mixed drinks. Problem drinkers also take much larger sips of their drinks than do moderate drinkers. Actually, they *gulp* rather than sip. The average sip for excessive drinkers is within the range of ½ ounce to 1¼ ounces. Moderate drinkers take an average of ⅕ to less than ½ ounce per sip. In some of my research studies I have observed heavy drinkers consistently consume an average of over 2 ounces per sip of straight Bourbon!

Heavy drinkers also drink alcoholic beverages about three times as fast as moderate drinkers. A *controlled* drinker might consume an 8-ounce glass of Scotch and water in 30 minutes, whereas an *uncontrolled* drinker would take only about 10

159

minutes. At that rate he would drink two to three times the number of drinks that the moderate drinker would in the same space of time. The moderate drinker is better able to pace himself. This is probably one of the important reasons why he is a *moderate drinker!*

The total time to consume a drink depends not only on the size of your sips (or gulps!) but also on the time intervals between your sips and between your drinks. Heavy drinkers vary the time interval between sips depending on what they are drinking. When they are drinking mixed drinks, their rate is quite fast. When drinking straight drinks or beer, they actually allow slightly more time between sips than moderate drinkers. However, their gulps are so large that they end up finishing their drinks faster.

Heavy drinkers also take very little time *between drinks.* While a moderate drinker might wait 10 to 20 minutes between drinks, his heavy-drinking buddy would be fixing another drink as soon as his last sip is finished. The heavy drinker may even be in the habit of filling up his drink with extra booze when it's only half empty.

In addition to these differences in drinking style, a problem drinker is less able to judge accurately the effects of alcohol on his system. That is, he cannot tell how much he's had to drink or how intoxicated he is on the basis of bodily sensations alone. Light and moderate drinkers are much more adept at this skill. These intriguing differences between heavy and moderate drinkers were determined in a series of studies in which drinkers were asked to estimate their own blood/alcohol level after consuming alcoholic beverages.

In these studies, research subjects drank alcohol in a disguised form, so that they were unable to tell what or how much they were drinking. Actually, they were given about an ounce of pure alcohol mixed with fruit juice. After about 20 minutes they were asked to estimate their blood/alcohol level. Estimates were often made on an actual blood/alcohol scale expressed in terms of milligrams of alcohol per milliliters of blood. These blood/alcohol levels are usually converted into a percentage, so that .01 percent indicates one mg per 100 ml. Generally, .00 percent indicates complete sobriety, and .25 percent indicates extreme intoxication bordering on loss of consciousness. In most states in our country a person would be considered too intoxicated to drive if his level were .10 percent or higher.

After the estimate was made, an alcohol breath test was administered to determine the exact blood/alcohol level. After a number of these estimates an average error or deviation score was calculated.

Light and moderate social drinkers usually have an average discrepancy score of about .02 percent. Actually, this is a very accurate estimate. Alcoholics have an average discrepancy score of about .11 percent. This is an extremely significant error in judgment.

Overweight individuals also exhibit differences in eating style when compared to individuals of normal weight. The similarities to those just discussed for heavy versus moderate drinkers are astounding. These similarities help to solidify the case for one general approach to addictive behaviors. Just as heavy drinkers consume straight as opposed to mixed drinks, overweight individuals eat more high-calorie foods (particularly those high in carbohydrates—that is, sweets and starches) than normal-weight individuals. In addition, they take larger mouthfuls of food. That is, they put more on their forks or spoons than normal-weight persons. They also do not chew their food as long and take a shorter time between bites. Generally, they finish their meals in about half the time of those who have better control over their eating.

While there have been fewer behavioral studies on smoking style, it appears that heavy smokers may smoke differently from light smokers. Heavy smokers consume a pack and a half or more per day, while light smokers consume an average of half a pack or less per day. It may be that heavy smokers smoke a more potent cigarette (in terms of tar and nicotine content), take longer drags, allow a shorter time between puffs, smoke a cigarette in a shorter period of time, and allow a shorter time between cigarettes.

What Do These Differences Mean?

Differences in response style indicate that the heavy smoker, drinker, and eater have less control over their habits. The drinker's and eater's response styles are particularly self-defeating because of physiological reasons. Let's suppose you haven't eaten in a while and you are really hungry. You fix yourself a good-sized meal, and, in your typical style, you eat very rapidly. You have finished your entire meal in about ten minutes. Now, from a physiological standpoint, it takes your body about 20 minutes after you start eating to feel satisfied. While you have eaten as much as you need in order to satisfy your hunger, your brain has not as yet received the message that you are "full." Therefore, after 10 minutes of eating you are still likely to feel hungry. As a result of your rapid eating style you may decide to have a second helping, perhaps a large second helping. After 10 more minutes you may begin to feel satisfied. Unfortunately, after 15 minutes more you may feel stuffed, since, physiologically, you have actually overeaten.

The same is true of the excessive drinker. You may feel like having a drink after a hard day at work. You may drink it so quickly, however, that even after you're finished you won't feel any effects. After another quick drink you not only start to feel relaxed but a little high. *Your drinking behavior is ahead of its effects on your system.* By the time you get to the third drink you are less likely to control further drinking because of your slightly intoxicated state.

Evaluating Your Personal Response Style—Self-Monitoring

The first step in changing your style of eating, drinking, or smoking is to evaluate the components of your behavior. For at least two or three days observe your response style and keep a written record of your behavior. You should evaluate at least three or more episodes. Therefore, if you only drink alcohol on two occasions per week, you should keep your records for a period of two weeks.

You will need to obtain a good sampling of your behavior in a variety of situations. Individual response styles vary quite a bit from situation to situation. For example, Jane finds that when she eats with other people, her response style is pretty good. She takes small bites, eats slowly, and takes about 20 minutes to eat her meal. In fact, the conversation with others helps to slow down the pace of her eating. When alone, however, she takes huge mouthfuls of food and finishes eating in about 5 minutes. If Jane had evaluated her eating style only during meals with other people, she might have concluded that her eating style was okay and no improvements were needed.

To evaluate your consumption style, refer to the behavioral components in Table 1. Since it would be very difficult to

Table 1 COMPONENTS OF CONSUMPTION STYLE

Substance	Potency	Absolute Amount Consumed	Amount per Mouthful	Time Between Mouthfuls	Time to Consume Substance	Time Between Episodes
Food	Nutritional quality (proteins, carbohydrates, fats)	Number of calories per day and number of separate eating episodes	Weight of mouthful; number of bites	Time between bites; chewing time	Time to complete meal	Time between meals or between eating episodes (including snacks)
Cigarettes	Tar and nicotine content	Number of cigarettes per day	Duration of puff; number of puffs	Time between puffs	Time to complete cigarette	Time between cigarettes
Alcohol	"Proof" or percentage of alcohol in beverage, and ratio of alcohol to mix	Number of ounces of alcohol per day or week	Ounces per sip; number of sips	Time between sips	Time to complete drink	Time between drinks or drinking episodes

observe all of these components simultaneously, pick two or three of the most important ones. If you're analyzing your smoking, you might choose (1) number of cigarettes per day, (2) number of puffs per cigarette, (3) time to finish cigarette, and (4) time between cigarettes. You can simplify your task by keeping a small index card or piece of paper between the cellophane wrapping and the paper container of your cigarette pack. Each time you light a cigarette jot down the time on the paper. By doing this you are keeping track of two components of your response style—the time between cigarettes and the number of cigarettes consumed. When you finish the cigarette, again write down the time next to the starting-time entry that you made for that cigarette. Finally, you can determine the number of puffs on a random basis. It is not likely that you will remember to count your puffs for each cigarette. Even if you do remember, you might have your mind on something else or you might be distracted because you're talking to someone else. If you end up counting the puffs for 25 percent of your cigarettes each day, you'll be doing fine.

It is helpful to enlist the aid of a spouse or good friend when monitoring your behavior. You might ask a specific person to count the number of puffs you take on at least three cigarettes during the day. This will give you an indication of any changes in your response style which occur when you are distracted by work or conversation. These observations by another person will also serve as a check on your own accuracy. Whether consciously or unconsciously, we all have a difficult time being completely objective about our own behavior.

When monitoring your eating style it is helpful to keep a notebook handy that will serve as your "eating diary." It will be easiest for you to record (1) number of calories per day,

(2) number of bites, (3) time between separate eating episodes, and (4) total time to consume a meal or snack. With all of your habit patterns, it would be almost impossible for you to calculate the amount per mouthful directly. Given the same quantity of food, cigarette, or alcohol at each episode, you could simply count the number of bites, puffs, or sips. The fewer the bites, for example, the more the amount per bite.

George is a forty-three-year-old group insurance agent working for a large national firm. He travels a great deal and often has to eat on the run. When he's at the office he usually grabs a quick bite at a nearby fast-food restaurant. His wife, Marge, loves to cook, and both she and George are each about 20 pounds overweight. George vows to lose his extra 20 pounds and decides, as a start, to keep track of his eating style for three days. He makes certain that he monitors his eating during a typical week in his life so that he can obtain an accurate picture of his eating patterns. He buys a small notebook and also purchases a golfer's wrist counter to aid him in counting the number of bites he takes. He describes his plan to his family so they won't think he's flipped his lid when they see him calculate how long it takes him to eat his dinner! He also asks his wife to help by counting his bites and noting the time it takes him to eat during at least one meal per day. George realizes that it is very important for him not to try to change his style of eating during this time. After three days of self-monitoring, George's notebook contains the entries illustrated in Table 2.

It is obvious that during George's eating episodes he takes only a few bites and eats very rapidly. For example, during lunch on the first day George finished a large hamburger in eight bites, taking only about 20 seconds between bites. This rapid eating pace may sound unbelievable to you until you

Table 2 GEORGE'S EATING STYLE

Meal	No. of Calories	No. of Bites	Average Time Between Bites	Total Time to Eat Meal or Snack
Breakfast				
2 eggs	140	18	10 sec.	7 min.
2 pieces of toast	130			
Coffee (black)	0			
Lunch				
Hamburger	561	8	20 sec.	5 min.
Soft drink	73			
Snack				
Candy bar at office	198	3	10 sec.	30 sec.
Dinner				
2 pork chops	764			
1 cup applesauce	116			
1 cup mashed potatoes	180			
1 cup string beans	30	40	25 sec.	15 min.
Large slice of cheesecake	325			
Coffee	0			
Snack				
20 potato chips	228			
Baloney sandwich	230	45	15 sec.	10 min.
Soft drink	73			

examine your own eating habits. George was astounded. He was especially surprised, as are most people, to find out that he was completely finished with most meals, even large ones, in 5 to 15 minutes. That's not enough time even to begin to enjoy eating.

As we look over Table 2 it is also evident that George consumed a great many foods that were not only high in calories but also high in carbohydrates and animal fat. His diet not only adds weight but also is unhealthy for him. To provide additional information George has asked his wife to record the number of chews and the time between bites two or three times during one of his meals. George finds out that on the average he chews each mouthful only five or six times. Also, he eats very rapidly, taking only a few seconds between mouthfuls. In fact, most of the time George is filling his mouth with a new forkful while he is still chewing food from the previous one.

Remember, when evaluating your response style, always

Break your habit down into its component parts.
Observe your behavior for a number of days.
Write down your responses on an index card.
Ask another person to observe your behavior at periodic intervals.

Changing Your Response Style

Now that you've determined exactly what your response style is, you are ready to modify your habits. Without this initial base-line evaluation you would not have been able to know exactly what changes were needed. In addition, you now have a starting point from which you can compare changes that you make. In this way you'll be better able to evaluate the progress of your Personal Habit Control plan.

The self-monitoring procedure you have just completed is actually one method of changing habits. You may have noticed that just by becoming more aware of your response style you started to change it. One well-known principle in behavioral psychology is that a behavior pattern will change merely through increased awareness of that habit. It is very likely that when you keep a written record of your drinking you'll find that your drinking decreases. Also, by self-monitoring your sip amount you'll automatically find that you begin to take smaller sips. Therefore, you have already modified your habits without realizing it.

Changes occuring as the result of self-awareness, however, are frequently smaller than the ones you will need to make. Without practicing a new response style consistently these changes will be short-lived.

Practice, feedback, and self-reward are all required to change consumption style permanently. It is best to start out slowly and change only one or two behavioral components at a time. If you try to change every aspect of your eating, drinking, or smoking style, you'll become confused and frustrated and give up.

By looking over your self-monitoring records you'll be able to tell what behaviors you need to change. In our earlier example, George might choose to work on slowing down the time between mouthfuls of food and taking smaller bites.

We'll discuss specific ways of modifying each of the response-style components listed in Table 1.

Substance Quality and Potency

It is very essential that you change the *quality* and/or *potency* of the substances you consume. For eating habits, this means changing the nutritional value of foods you eat. Many calorie booklets and labels on packaged foods include nutritional information on the protein, carbohydrate, and fat content of the foods you eat. Generally, you need a balance of these three nutritional units in your diet.

The simplest diet, and one that most frequently leads to *permanent* weight control, is one that reduces your over-all caloric intake without sacrificing a good nutritional balance. Diets that emphasize one type of food, such as grapefruit or bananas, or fasting programs in which you give up all solid foods, do change the quality of what you eat. After these diets are over, you'll most probably go back to your previous high-calorie foods.

In my current obesity program we use a very low-calorie— 700 a day—diet that is nutritionally well balanced with 60 grams of proteins, 60 grams of carbohydrates, and 25 grams of fat. This dietary program is low in animal fat, not merely to reduce calories but also to reduce cholesterol and triglycerides, two types of fatty deposits that collect in the blood vessels and apparently contribute to hypertension, stroke, and heart disease. With this nutritionally well-balanced diet, once an individual has attained an ideal weight he can simply increase the number of calories he consumes but maintain the same qualitative balance. Therefore, during the diet process he is learning to control the quality of his food intake, which in turn becomes a permanent habit pattern.

Food content and quality can effect how hungry you feel. For example, foods that are high in carbohydrates (sugar or starches) will immediately raise your blood sugar level. However, your body will compensate for this by secreting insulin. In overweight individuals an overabundance of insulin is secreted, which within two to three hours reduces your blood sugar *below* its normal level. Very low blood sugar levels are often associated with feelings of hunger. Therefore, a quick candy bar pick-me-up in the middle of the day may temporarily increase your energy level, but it also may increase your feelings of hunger later that afternoon.

A good example of this phenomenon is provided by Melanie. Melanie is a twenty-three-year-old school teacher who lives alone. She never eats breakfast, since she is always getting up late. She usually has a cup of coffee in the teacher's lounge at school. She wants to lose a few pounds and develop better eating habits, so she decides to eat three well-balanced meals a day. On the first day of her new eating pattern she gets up early and has a glass of orange juice, three pieces of toast, and coffee. After breakfast she feels full and satisfied. At about 10 A.M. she begins to feel extremely hungry. She is craving food. She can't understand this feeling, because she has eaten breakfast. In fact, she never experienced such mid-morning hunger when she only had coffee for breakfast. As a result of this experience Melanie decides to go back to her old eating patterns.

What happened? Melanie was the victim of a carbohydrate-insulin-induced drop in her blood sugar level which occurred about two hours after eating. Her breakfast was full of carbohydrates—sugar in the orange juice and starches in the toast. If she had eaten a high-protein breakfast—one egg or certain types of cereal—she would have continued to feel satisfied throughout the morning. Proteins exercise a longer-lasting effect on hunger.

A general suggestion regarding changes in your dietary patterns is to choose a low-calorie diet that provides an adequate balance of carbohydrates, proteins, and fats. Certainly you should consult your physician before beginning a diet. Beware of most diet books on the market. Most stress quick weight loss at the expense of good nutrition. You will never succeed with most of these approaches.

Changing the quality or potency of your cigarettes is a relatively simple matter. Cigarette brands now list the tar and nicotine content on the package. These might vary from 27 mg tar and 1.7 mg nicotine to approximately 1 mg tar and 0.1

mg nicotine per cigarette. Simply compare brands and try out a variety of cigarettes that are significantly lower in tar and nicotine than your current brand.

Modifying the potency of alcohol is also a relatively straight-forward proposition. Alcohol potency is determined by (1) the alcoholic content of the beverage itself and (2) the ratio of alcohol to mix in preparing a drink. You can determine the alcoholic content of beer, wine, or liquor by its "proof." Alcoholic content equals half the value of the "proof" on the label. Eighty-proof Bourbon contains 40 percent alcohol. The alcohol content of commonly used alcoholic beverages is as follows:

Beverage	Percentage of Alcohol
Bourbon, Scotch, gin, etc.	40–50
Beer	4–6
Wine	12–14
Cocktail wine (sherry)	20
Liqueurs	30–60

A standard alcoholic drink is usually considered to be the amount of beverage that contains ½ ounce of pure alcohol. On the basis of this standard, one 4-ounce glass of wine, one 12-ounce can of beer, and one ounce of whiskey would all contain the same amount of alcohol. Most people find this difficult to believe. According to this standard, ten beers are as potent as 10 ounces of gin. This does not mean, however, that you will become as intoxicated on beer or wine as you do on Bourbon or Scotch. First of all, your typical drink may contain 1½ to 2 ounces of Scotch mixed with water, which would be equivalent to two beers. Second, you might drink these beverages at a different rate. It would probably take you longer to drink 12 ounces of beer than it would one ounce of vodka.

In terms of alcohol content *per se,* beer and wine would be less potent than whiskey. There is no appreciable difference among different liquors. To modify potency, then, you may decide to switch from liquor to wine and beer, or from a 100-proof to an 80-proof Bourbon. Remember, however, that quantity can more than offset changes in quality. If you switch from one 2-ounce vodka and tonic each evening to four beers, you're worse off than when you started.

One further aspect of potency, as far as some alcoholic beverages are concerned, is the ratio of liquor to mix for each drink. When drinking Bourbon, Scotch, gin, or vodka, *never* drink a straight, nonmixed drink. Also, avoid the more potent cocktails, such as martinis and Manhattans, which mix one alcoholic beverage with another. Get into the habit of calculating the ratio of alcohol to mix; *always* use a shot glass or some type of measuring glass so that you know exactly how many ounces of alcohol you have in the drink. If you generally mix a drink consisting of 2 ounces of Scotch with 2 ounces of water, either decrease the Scotch or increase the water content of each drink. You can also do both. It might help to start this process gradually—to wean yourself from potent drinks. Set a new goal for yourself each week. During one week every drink you make yourself might have 1½ ounces (one shot) of Bourbon to 2 ounces of water. The next week you might mix a 1:3 ratio of Bourbon to water.

Finally, avoid carbonated mixers, such as club soda or cola. Alcohol mixed with carbonated beverages enters your bloodstream at a more rapid rate than when you mix it with a noncarbonated beverage.

In making changes in the quality and potency of your food, alcohol, and cigarettes, you must be aware of certain negative side effects that might occur in your response style. In one of my experiments on drinking patterns, my colleagues and I were examining the relationships among the behavioral components of drinking. We were particularly interested in the effects of changes in one component of response style on other components.

In our laboratory we set up a simulated living room setting, complete with alcoholic beverages and mixers. We could observe the setting via closed-circuit television from an adjacent room. We enlisted the assistance of a number of problem drinkers and asked them, one by one, to sit in this room and drink. Needless to say, we had more than enough volunteers! As each volunteer consumed the alcohol, we observed and calculated the ratio of alcoholic beverage to mix used for each drink, the average amount consumed per sip, the average time between sips, and the number of sips.

During the second phase of the study we asked each volunteer to modify one component of drinking style. When these problem drinkers changed from straight drinks (that is, Bourbon alone) to mixed drinks (that is, 50 percent Bourbon and 50 percent water in each drink), drastic changes in other drinking components were observed. Almost immediately they started taking much larger sips. One subject began drinking almost an ounce per sip! In addition, they drank much more rapidly—almost twice as fast as before. In a sense they were compensating for the change. Interestingly enough, none of the drinkers was aware that the change in potency had affected the other aspects of his or her drinking.

You must keep this interaction in mind when changing your response style. In fact, you must change *every* component discussed in this chapter or you may be learning a different but equally inappropriate consumption style. You may end up smoking a low-tar and -nicotine cigarette but inhaling much more deeply during each puff than you did with your previous brand. You may take smaller bites of food but eat at a faster rate. Unless you are willing to change your total response style, don't even begin to change it at all. You may develop a more detrimental behavior pattern than the one you started with.

Absolute Amount Consumed

In addition to potency, you must also change the total amount that you consume of a substance at any given time. In fact, this is really your ultimate goal, and the changes you make in the other components will help you attain this goal. However, you can also decrease your total consumption in a direct way.

This is a very simple procedure. You merely set an absolute limit for yourself. When changing eating patterns, set a limit on the number of calories you will allow yourself each day. Most diets allow about 1,000 to 1,500 calories. Under medical supervision, you may decide to set a lower limit than this. By continuing your eating diary, you can keep track of all calories consumed each day. Self-monitoring is a *must* to insure changes in amount consumed. It is very easy to fool yourself if you're not counting calories and writing them down.

If you are trying to moderate your drinking, you can put a limit on the number of drinks (remember, this means one beer, one glass of wine, or one ounce of liquor) per day or week or the number of ounces of alcohol consumed. If you measure each drink on the basis of the standard drink as we are defining it here, you can simply limit total drinks con-sumed. If you limit drinks, however, you may find yourself sticking to your limit but making more potent drinks. In this case you'd have to set a limit in terms of ounces, or at least be aware of your tendency to cheat. In this regard, you should always use a shot glass and at the end of each day write down the number and type of drinks consumed. If you drink mostly at home, keep your "drinking diary" in the liquor cabinet and record each drink as you prepare it. When self-recording any behavior, it is most helpful to write it down *before* you eat, drink, or smoke. Writing this information beforehand helps you to rethink your decision to "fill your mouth" and often prevents an episode of consumption.

With drinking, it is sometimes more helpful to set a limit on the number of drinks per episode than per day or week. This is especially true if you drink mostly at parties and small social gatherings. A good rule of thumb is to set two or three drinks as your limit at a party. Before you even get to the party you should plan how many drinks you'll have.

Planning is an important aspect of limiting your consump-tion. You should plan your meals so that you know at the beginning of each week what meals you will have, with the number of calories in each. If you know you'll be going to a dinner party on Thursday evening, plan the rest of your day accordingly. Eat about half as many calories for breakfast and lunch that day, since you'll probably be eating more than usual at the dinner party. You can also have a weekly drink plan and cigarette plan.

Your cigarette plan should consist of limiting the number of cigarettes for each day or each occasion. If you're going to a party, set a limit of, let's say, five cigarettes for the evening. Bring only five cigarettes with you. Accessibility is a major factor in overconsumption. If more food, drink, or cigarettes are readily available than your limit, you'll have a very difficult time. You can insure against your cadging cigarettes by telling everyone at the party that you're cutting down your smoking and have set a limit for your consumption that evening.

Amount per Mouthful

One method of modifying your total consumption and rate of consumption is to decrease the size of your bites, puffs, and sips. You can tell how badly you need to change this component by referring to your self-evaluation record. When you were monitoring your response style, did you find that you took very few bites during a meal, or very few puffs on your cigarette? This probably means that your bites or puffs are much too large.

Unfortunately, it is extremely impractical to calculate the amount you consume per mouthful exactly. You're not going to weigh each forkful or measure each sip. You can, however, strive to take smaller bites, sips, or puffs than you did during your previous meal, drink, or cigarette.

The easiest method of reducing amount per mouthful is simply to increase the total number of bites per meal, sips per drink, and puffs per cigarette. Remember, when you are comparing the number of mouthfuls from episode to episode, make certain that the total amount of substance that you consumed is approximately the same on both occasions. Otherwise increases in number of mouthfuls may be meaningless. Ten drags on a king-size cigarette are not better than seven on a regular one. Amount consumed per puff may be equally high for both.

Since there are no specific norms for this behavioral component of habit style, it is difficult to provide you with an ultimate goal. Generally, however, you should strive for five or more small bites per minute while eating. You should not inhale during each puff on a cigarette any longer than *two seconds*. In addition, strive for *eight* or more small puffs per cigarette.

As far as drinking is concerned, your ultimate goal should be to take less than ½ ounce per sip of an alcoholic beverage. This would mean sixteen or more sips for an 8-ounce drink. A 4-ounce glass of wine should be consumed in about ten sips.

One very good way to slow down the pace of your consumption is to lengthen the time between mouthfuls. That is, take a longer time between puffs, bites, and sips.

This is really a lot more difficult than it sounds. In fact, this style component is one of the most difficult to change. The old "hand to mouth" routine is so automatic that your hand will fill your mouth before you realize what has happened. You must not only be aware of approximately how much time elapses between mouthfuls but, more important, you must plan to bridge that gap of time with an alternative behavior.

First of all, find out what you're doing between mouthfuls. While eating you're probably holding your fork or spoon, waiting to finish chewing the last mouthful. Some people even begin to load up the fork immediately after each previous mouthful. To be successful at increasing this bite-to-bite time interval, you must *put your fork or spoon down on your plate after each bite*. That's right, get your hand off it! You must practice letting go of your fork at every meal. Then rate yourself on the percentage of bites after which you put your fork down on your plate.

Another method of slowing down time between mouthfuls is to increase your chewing time. More chewing not only assists the digestive process but also slows the pace of eating; generally you should take at least ten chews or more per bite. Your new routine should include (1) taking a small mouthful of food, (2) putting your fork down on the plate, and (3) chewing your food slowly and carefully (at least ten times). After swallowing the food you should wait a few seconds before picking up your fork for the next mouthful.

Imagine that you're a gourmet and your job is to savor each mouthful and then rate its taste. To do this you must chew very slowly and then take a few seconds to think about the taste. One good rule of thumb is *never* to put any food into your mouth until at least three seconds after you have swallowed the previous mouthful of food.

Time intervals between puffs of a cigarette and sips of a drink are just as important. When smoking, try to put your cigarette in an ashtray between puffs. If that's not possible, switch it to your other hand. When you're ready for another puff, return the cigarette to your dominant hand. Both of these maneuvers will slow you down. Try the same procedures while drinking: put your drink down or hold it in your other hand. Keep your hands busy between puffs or sips. Try fiddling with your keys, a pen, or worry beads. If you find yourself going for another puff or sip, clench your fist to remind yourself to wait. Remember to clench the fist that doesn't contain the cigarette or drink! On second thought, that might be an excellent method of habit control—destroying the substance before it gets to your mouth!

In terms of specific time standards, you should try to allow at least 1 to 1½ minutes between puffs of a cigarette, 2 minutes or more between sips of an alcoholic beverage, and about

30 seconds or more between bites of food. These intervals are measured from the time a mouthful enters your mouth until the next mouthful is put to your lips.

Total Time to Consume a Substance

If you modify all the components described above, you will have increased the total time it takes you to consume each cigarette, meal, or drink. Just as a check on yourself, however, you may wish to keep track of the total time of consumption. If so, you should allow at least 20 minutes for each meal. Anything less than that is too fast. It should take you at least 6 to 8 minutes to smoke a cigarette. Drinking time will vary depending on the beverage and how much is available. You should strive for 30 to 45 minutes for each 8-ounce glass of liquor and mix or 12-ounce can of beer.

If you're not taking this long to consume a substance, evaluate your response style. What component are you disregarding? Checking your total consumption time on a periodic basis is an excellent method of evaluating your response-style changes.

Time Interval Between Episodes

Generally speaking, you should eat three well-balanced meals per day, with meals spaced about 4 to 6 hours apart. The time interval between cigarettes can be very individualized and is related to the total number of cigarettes you allow yourself on a particular day. If you've vowed to smoke only five cigarettes, you might want to space them out evenly over the day with about 2 to 3 hours between cigarettes. When at a party, you may decide to smoke them about 30 minutes apart. It is good to decide on a time interval and then stick to it. At home, after each smoke you can set a timer or alarm clock to go off at the proper time for your next cigarette. The situation is the same for drinking. Time between drinks depends on the number of drinks you have allotted yourself. Since alcohol is used up by your body at the rate of about one ounce per hour, you should drink accordingly to avoid intoxication. After each drink you may wish to wait 20 minutes before fixing another. At a party or small get-together, a good idea would be to fix yourself a nonalcoholic beverage between alcoholic drinks. During an evening you should alternate between alcoholic and nonalcoholic beverages. In fact, it might be best to make your very first drink a nonalcoholic one. After you reach your drinking limit, drink only nonalcoholic beverages. By always having a drink handy, you also avoid being pressured to have another drink (the alcoholic kind) by your friendly host or hostess.

How to Control Habits Through Bodily Sensations

If you are a heavy consumer of food or alcohol, your best method of control is through the modification of *external* factors associated with eating and drinking. These include the behavioral components of your response style which have been outlined in this chapter.

As an additional control mechanism you may also want to develop *internal* control. Since many of you are deficient in such control (as described earlier in this chapter), it may be very difficult or impossible for you to regulate your behavior based on "true" hunger or blood/alcohol level. For maximum insurance, however, you should learn to rely on as many control mechanisms as you can.

As you change your eating patterns and begin to lose

weight, you'll notice that you also begin to feel hungry. I mean *really* hungry. These hunger feelings may be different from the ones you're used to. These feelings are actually true physiological hunger. You haven't experienced them in a long time, since you've never given your body a chance to be without food long enough to be hungry. The hunger you've experienced before is psychological rather than physical hunger. Don't be disturbed by these new feelings. Actually, you should rejoice. Your body is working again. You can take this opportunity to learn what true hunger actually feels like. Then you can begin to condition yourself to eat only in response to physiological hunger. Get in touch with your feelings of hunger. Become aware of them. Think about the sounds your stomach is making. Experience the "empty" feeling in your stomach. Each time you get this feeling, concentrate on what is going on inside you. Through this self-awareness process you will gradually learn what bodily hunger really means.

The same procedures, only perhaps on a more sophisticated level, can be used to learn to estimate your blood/alcohol level. Table 3 represents a drinking scale to help you learn what bodily sensations are usually associated with certain blood/alcohol levels. Remember that the number of drinks needed for you to reach a particular blood/alcohol level will vary, particularly according to weight. If you weigh 240 pounds, your blood/alcohol level would be approximately .03 percent after consuming 2 drinks in one hour. If you weigh 160 pounds, it would be .05 percent. The table is general enough, however, so that you'll be able to use it to judge your blood/alcohol level. Table 4 will give you an indication of the relationship between blood/alcohol level and body weight.

The next time you have a drink that is measured carefully (that is, 4 ounces of wine, a 12-ounce can of beer, or one

Table 3 DRINKING SCALE

*Percent of Blood/Alcohol Concentration**	
0–0.03 (1–2 drinks)	No significant effects on behavior, but possible lightness in the head and slight feelings of warmth
0.04–0.06 (2–3 drinks)	Feelings of warmth and relaxation, feeling less socially inhibited, increased talkativeness, "tingling" sensations
0.07–0.10 (4–6 drinks)	Marked relaxation and warmth, clumsiness, slowed reaction time, numbness
0.11–0.14 (7–9 drinks)	Marked clumsiness, slowed reaction time, judgment impaired
0.15–0.20 (10 or more)	Marked intoxication, coordination impaired, staggering

* Blood/alcohol concentration refers to milligrams of alcohol per 100 milliliters of blood. For example, .10 percent is equal to a concentration of 100 mg percent.

Table 4 APPROXIMATE BLOOD/ALCOHOL PERCENTAGE

Drinks	Body Weight in Pounds								
	100	120	140	160	180	200	220	240	*Influenced rarely*
1	.04	.03	.03	.02	.02	.02	.02	.02	
2	.08	.06	.05	.05	.04	.04	.03	.03	
3	.11	.09	.08	.07	.06	.06	.05	.05	
4	.15	.12	.11	.09	.08	.08	.07	.06	
5	.19	.16	.13	.12	.11	.09	.09	.08	*Possibly*
6	.23	.19	.16	.14	.13	.11	.10	.09	
7	.26	.22	.19	.16	.15	.13	.12	.11	
8	.30	.25	.21	.19	.17	.15	.14	.13	*Definitely*
9	.34	.28	.24	.21	.19	.17	.15	.14	
10	.38	.31	.27	.23	.21	.19	.17	.16	

One drink equals 1 ounce of 80-proof liquor or 12 ounces of beer. Subtract .01 percent for each 40 minutes of drinking.

ounce of 80-proof liquor with a mixer), concentrate on your bodily sensations as you drink. After you've finished, what are you feeling? You may feel slightly relaxed and warm. If you are a very large person, you may feel nothing. If you weigh 120 pounds or less you may feel very relaxed and talkative. Use Table 3 to match your feelings with your blood/alcohol level. Now have another drink. Again concentrate on your feelings. Do you feel very relaxed? Are you becoming less socially inhibited? Continue drinking until you reach a level between .07 and .10 percent. What is happening now? Concentrate on any feelings of numbness or tingling sensations in your face, hands, or arms. Are you getting clumsy? Is your speech slurred?

Repeat this procedure several times over the next few weeks. Try to use a combination of the guidelines in Table 4, relating weight to blood/alcohol level, and your own internal feelings. A good level of control of drinking is achieved by never exceeding the .04–.06 percent blood/alcohol-level range.

How to Make Sure That Changes Occur

Changing components of your response style may not be as easy as it seems. One reason is that you've had so much practice at your old habits that you will automatically and, without your awareness, resist change. If you are forty years of age you've eaten well over 40,000 meals using your old response style. That would be like trying to change your golf stroke after hitting the ball the same way 40,000 times. This style of your habit pattern has been so well conditioned that you will have to actively modify your behavior. Merely reading this chapter and giving some thought to your response style will be of little value. But if you work diligently on the changes outlined so far, and stick to them faithfully for a few weeks, your *new* response style will become as automatic as your old one. After a while you will no longer have to think about the number of bites you take or the time it takes you to drink an alcoholic beverage. You will have taught yourself a new habit pattern that will become a permanent part of your behavior.

Reminding Yourself to Remember

You may notice that even when you are very sincere about changing your response style, you may simply forget occasionally. You must remember, however, that every time you forget, every time you smoke, drink, or eat in your old way, it will take a longer time for your new style to become automatic.

You may find that you are almost finished with a meal or a cigarette before you remember about changing your pattern of consumption. There are several ways to counteract this difficulty. It is helpful to use visual cues to remind yourself. For example, keep a small sign by your place setting at the table which might say, "Are you taking smaller bites?" or "Don't forget! *Personal Habit Control* during every meal." If you're a smoker, the smoking-diary card you keep in your cigarette package will remind you. You may also remember to change your style of smoking by keeping your cigarettes in a place different from your customary one. When you reach for a cigarette in your usual pocket and remember that you now keep them elsewhere, you'll also remember your new habit-control plan. You might try buying a distinctive cigarette case as a visual reminder.

If you are a drinker, place a small sign in your liquor cabinet or on your bar saying, "Think before you drink!"

It may help to have a close friend or relative remind you of your new plan when you are about to smoke, drink, or eat. Some of you may resent this procedure and regard it as annoying. If so, don't use it. Otherwise ask someone to remind you discreetly (perhaps with a nonverbal gesture—a wink, for example) at appropriate times to control your response style.

Evaluating Your Progress and Achieving Your Goals

An extremely important element of successful behavior change is setting specific behavioral goals for yourself. Each day or each week you should be actively trying to change a particular component or set of components in your response style. In the beginning, goals should be set in relation to your initial evaluation of your response style. If your typical pattern is to chew each mouthful of food about 5 times, don't try to achieve 20 chews per mouthful the first week. Be more realistic. The biggest mistake most people make is to be overly ambitious in changing their habits. Remember that it took many, many years to develop your habits. Take a little time to develop new ones. During the first week of your new program you should strive for an average of 10 chews per mouthful. Of course this will just be an average during an entire meal. Don't proceed to your next goal on this component until you have successfully achieved the 10-chews-per-mouthful goal on at least three consecutive days. This is very important in the development of a new pattern. If you have difficulty with the 10-chews goal, drop back to 7 or 8 chews. Use the same system for other components with all of your habits.

When attempting to set specific goals, analyze yourself. Are you the kind of person who usually sets very high goals, which, perhaps, you seldom attain? Or do you set goals that are actually lower than your capabilities? This self-analysis will help you better evaluate the behavioral habit-change goals you set. One very helpful way of evaluating the appropriateness of your goals is through a rating system. Let's suppose that you promise yourself to faithfully practice (1) drinking less potent drinks and (2) limiting yourself to two alcoholic beverages per day. This is your goal for the next week. Now ask yourself, on a scale of 1 to 10, "How likely am I to accomplish this goal?" On this scale 1 indicates very little likelihood and 10 indicates a 100 percent certainty. If you give a rating of 8, 9, or 10, that's fine. Stick to the goal you've set. If you give a rating of 7 or less, you may be setting yourself up for failure. By this rating you're already telling yourself that your chances are poor. This self-defeating attitude will get you every time. If your rating is low, reconsider it and ask, "What goal would I be able to achieve with a high degree of certainty?" In evaluating your drinking goal you may find that one of the reasons for your low rating is that you know this will be a particularly stressful week. Perhaps you've been invited to a couple of cocktail parties and you're worried about keeping your resolve in that atmosphere. That's perfectly natural. Just modify your goal a little bit. Change your goal so that you'll (1) drink less potent drinks, and (2) limit yourself to two alcoholic beverages a day on at least four of seven days next week. Again, rate your goal on the 1 to 10 scale. You may now find that you have given a rating of 9 and feel very positive about your chances of success. If your rating is still low, reevaluate your goal once again.

If you continue to give low ratings, you may have to examine your attitude rather than your goal. Because of years of trying and failing at changing your habits, you may have developed a negative attitude toward your chances of succeeding. If this is your feeling, give yourself and this new system a chance. Since we are dealing with one component of your behavior at a time, the task of changing should not seem so overwhelming. Success at changing one component of your response style will help you develop a more positive attitude about changing other aspects of your behavior pattern. Rather than sitting around waiting for your attitude to improve, start changing your behavior. That's right—even if you don't really believe it will work. Because if you start out with small goals, it *will* work. Then behavior change will result in attitude change.

After setting your goals, you must have some way to evaluate them. This process of feedback on the extent of your behavior change is absolutely essential. You must have a systematic method of judging your success. Your eating, smoking, or drinking diary is the basis for evaluating your efforts. If you continue to record the components of your response style during your behavior-change efforts, you'll have a running account of your accomplishments. This also places the emphasis of your evaluation on comparisons between your present and past behavior on a day-to-day basis—that is, how you did today as compared to yesterday. Avoid comparing your progress with that of somebody else. You should be concerned only with your own progress as it relates to your own past performance.

You should examine the results of your behavior-change efforts at the end of each day or even at the end of each episode of consumption. For example, as you complete each meal, cigarette, or drink, fill out an evaluation form on yourself. This form might resemble the one presented in Table 5. You could fill this form out in several ways. Merely place a "Yes" or "No" next to each component based on your efforts

Table 5

Date	Breakfast	Lunch	Dinner
Smaller bites			
More time between bites			
Put fork or spoon down between bites			
20 minutes or more to consume meal			

during breakfast, lunch, and dinner. You may want to give yourself partial credit for remembering to take smaller bites about half of the time. In this case, use percentages for feedback to indicate the percentage of times you modified a component of response style during each meal. For example, on 50 percent of your mouthfuls you took smaller bites, on 75 percent of your opportunities you put your fork down between bites, and so on. This immediate feedback on your performance will keep your motivation high and speed up the process of behavior change. It will also help you evaluate your progress and establish new goals for yourself..

In setting goals for your habit change program

1. Be realistic and specific.
2. Rate your chances of success.
3. Evaluate your goals and modify them.
4. Give yourself credit when you succeed.

CHAPTER EIGHT

How to Help Your Family and Friends Help You

Several years ago Dr. Alan Marlatt, a well-known behavioral scientist at the University of Washington, wanted to find out why people reverted to old habits after successfully controlling them for a period of time. He was particularly interested in studying the specific circumstances that trigger episodes of excessive drinking. After an extensive analysis of numerous events reported by problem drinkers to set off their drinking, he narrowed his search to two primary targets. In nearly 60 percent of all problem drinkers interviewed, over-consumption of alcohol was preceded by (1) a feeling of frustration and the inability to express anger, and (2) social pressure from "friends" to have a drink. Ex-smokers and dieters who return to their old habit patterns report the same phenomena. Other people who frustrate you or who goad you into overconsumption are really your "friendly enemies." The friend who urges you to have "one little" smoke, drink, or bite may be thought of as a *pusher,* similar to a dealer pushing heroin on his prey.

The case of Walter Martin provides a good example. Walter is a forty-six-year-old attorney who works for an agency of the federal government. During his annual physical exam his blood pressure was 180/90. Blood-pressure readings were taken by his doctor over the next few days, and they remained high. Walter's doctor prescribed medication and advised him to lose 20 pounds and quit smoking or risk a stroke or heart attack. Walter was very concerned, especially since his father had died of a heart attack at an early age. He vowed to improve his health. He took his medication faithfully, started an exercise and jogging program, became more calorie-conscious, and quit smoking.

Unfortunately, within six months Walter was smoking again —in fact, more than he had smoked before. To make clear what happened I'll have to tell you a little more about Walter and his life. Walter is married, with two teenage children. He is a fairly well-adjusted individual who feels most comfortable when his life is well ordered. He dislikes conflicts, especially with his family or close friends. He is often described by others as a "really great guy" who would do anything to help his friends. Walter likes other people and often goes out of his way not to offend anyone.

Six months after he had quit smoking Walter acquired a new boss. His new superior was a mediocre attorney who had climbed the administrative hierarchy in the federal government as the result of two "qualifications": (1) he happened to have been around longer than anybody else, and (2) he never "made waves." He was frequently chosen for administrative posts because he was a safe, noncontroversial choice. He spent most of his time doing as little as possible and giving most of his own work to his subordinates, including Walter. When Walter was unable to complete both his own assignments and those of his boss, he was reprimanded. On the day of his reprimand Walter was understandably upset. He was extremely frustrated and angry. He felt unable to express his anger for fear of repercussions. He had seen his boss make life very uncomfortable for one of his colleagues. Besides, Walter was next in line for his boss's job and didn't want to jeopardize his chances for promotion. That afternoon Walter was describing his situation to several peers. All of his friends were smoking and drinking coffee at the time. One of the new attorneys, who was unaware of Walter's no-smoking campaign, offered him a cigarette. Walter hesitantly refused. Another friend said, "Aw, come on, Walter, you're upset and mad as hell. A cigarette will calm your nerves." Another friend held out a cigarette. Well, to make a long story short, Walter took the cigarette and lit up.

The two precipitating events—unexpressed anger and social pressure—triggered off smoking. Perhaps if either event had occurred alone he could have resisted. Social pressure without a feeling of frustration might not have been difficult for him to handle. Also, if his friends hadn't been around to make smoking "easy" for him, he might have calmed down enough by the next day to resist.

Social pressure to indulge in cigarettes, alcohol, or food is present all the time. In fact, most people's first smoking or drinking experience occurs as the direct result of encouragement and, perhaps, challenge from others. Remember your first cigarette or alcoholic beverage? If you're like most people, you probably were a teenager with a group of friends who were all "experimenting" and coaxing one another along. How could you refuse? To refuse would have meant social ostracism just at a time in your life when acceptance by your peers was essential. Anything was better than to be considered an oddball who wouldn't smoke and drink or, worse yet, to be thought of as "just a kid." And what made smoking and drinking even more exciting was that you knew your parents would object. What better way to assert your independence of family domination?

What You Are Up Against

There are several reasons why social pressure may be difficult for you. Perhaps such situations make you feel uncomfortable because of possible negative consequences of your refusal. All sorts of unpleasant outcomes of your saying "No" probably run through your mind. How many of the following thoughts are familiar to you?

"How can I refuse to drink with Jim? After all, he's been a good, steady customer for years. He *expects* me to drink with him. If I don't, it'll make him uncomfortable and I might lose his business."

"Marge went out of her way to make that dessert for me tonight. If I don't have some, it might really hurt her feelings. She's been upset lately, anyhow. I don't want to make things worse for her."

"I don't want to be a stick-in-the-mud tonight. What will my date think of me if I don't drink? He'll think I'm dull!"

Attitudes versus Behavior

There are actually two components of refusing offers of food, cigarettes, or alcohol. The first is the *attitude* you have about the appropriateness of refusing. The second is the actual *behavior* involved in refusing. Before you learn *how* to refuse we must examine *why* you should refuse.

Early in life you may have learned myths about your behavior in relation to others. *As part of your habit-change efforts you must be prepared to believe that*

1. You have a *right* to control your habits, and other people must respect that right.
2. You have a personal responsibility to defend your

rights by not allowing others to influence you
unduly.
3. You also have a responsibility to let people know
when they are interfering with your rights.
4. If, in the process of standing up for your rights,
other people become upset or get their feelings
hurt, that's *their* problem, not *your* problem.

People who are controlling their habits often feel intimidated when interacting with others who are not controlling their habits. The dieter feels compelled to apologize for not accepting offers of high-calorie foods. So-called "legitimate" reasons must be given for the refusal. Thus the ex-heavy drinker has to find an "acceptable" reason for refusing a drink, such as "I've been having trouble with my ulcer lately and my doctor advised me not to drink alcohol." Or a dieter often says, "I'm not supposed to have sweets," as if someone were imposing the restriction on him. Do not fall into this pattern. Take responsibility for yourself and your decision to change your habit. Be proud of the fact that you are controlling your habit. Be straightforward and say, "No, thank you, I have decided to cut down on my drinking." No reasons or excuses are necessary. Do other people explain to you why they're having dessert or a third drink or another cigarette? Certainly not. Then why do you feel so odd about refusing these things?

Refusal Training
The behavioral components of a refusal are relatively straightforward. The trick is to put them all together and use them skillfully. These components include both verbal and

nonverbal elements. That is, it's not just *what* you say that's important but *how* you say it. In fact the *how,* the nonverbal aspects of your behavior, are essential to an adequate refusal. Let's examine each component in detail.

NONCOMPLIANCE

The first and most obvious component of a refusal response is the expression of a negative statement of noncompliance. Use simple terms: say "No" or "No, thank you" or "I don't care for one." Your response should be direct and to the point. Do not beat around the bush. Statements such as "Well . . . ah . . . I don't think that I'd better have a cigarette" simply are too vague and leave you wide open for arguments geared toward talking you into having a cigarette. *Do not* complicate the matter by giving a lot of excuses for your refusal. A simple, "No, thanks" is sufficient.

There are, however, some circumstances in which you may wish to give a brief explanation for your refusal. For example, it is perfectly okay to say, "No, thanks, I have given up smoking." To a hostess offering dessert you might say, "Thank you, but your delicious meal was *more* than enough for me." While you also could add, "Besides, I'm watching my weight" or "I'm dieting," such explanations are really not necessary. The main reason for not relying on these statements is that you will *not* be dieting forever. You must think of these refusal skills as being *permanent;* that is, you must be able to refuse dessert, if you really don't want it, even when you're not on a diet. In the beginning of your habit-control plan you may be proud of your efforts and eager to share your new system with others. However, after a while you may become a bit tired of explaining your diet or why you're not drinking so much anymore. So if in the beginning you find it helpful to explain to people what you are doing, then do it. Just don't feel as though you *owe* them an explanation.

Unfortunately, heavy drinkers and alcoholics have an additional problem—the social stigma placed on their condition. An alcoholic is socially damned if he drinks, and damned if he doesn't. If he drinks at parties people say, "There he goes again—no willpower." If he refuses drinks they say, "He's not drinking at all tonight. I knew he was an alcoholic." He's stigmatized no matter what. I would not suggest lying about your reasons for drinking less or abstaining. Don't overexplain either. You might say, "No, thanks, I'm trying to drink less these days" or "Drinking is not good for my health." With close friends you may feel that you want to give more of a detailed explanation. You might say, "You know, Fred, I've been worried about my drinking lately. I've been drinking way too much, so I've decided not to drink tonight." With business associates or acquaintances such explanations are *not* necessary and would be considered by some to be inappropriate.

REQUESTING A CHANGE IN BEHAVIOR

If you are likely to have continued contact with someone over a period of time it is best to request a permanent change in their behavior toward you. For example, if you socialize with a certain friend quite a bit, you should request that he refrain from offering you certain foods, or alcohol, or cigarettes ever again. If you simply refuse with a brief explanation on one occasion, you'll have to go through the same explanation again and again. Simply say, "John, it would really help me out if you never offered me an alcoholic drink again." Such a statement conveys the message both to John and to yourself that you consider your new habit-control plan to be permanent. Therefore, you should also avoid statements that imply only temporary change, such as "I'd better not have a cigarette tonight" or "My doctor says I'd better lay off the booze for a while" or "I'd better not—I'm feeling a little sick to my stomach tonight." All remarks of this nature leave you open to offers of food, cigarettes, or alcohol on other occasions.

With a spouse you can be very specific and say, "It would really help me out if you just never offered me snacks again. If I want any, I'll get them myself. But let's have an agreement that you won't offer them to me now or ever."

OFFERING AN ALTERNATIVE

It is often helpful to add an offer of an alternative to your refusal. That is, you might request a diet soft drink or a club soda and lemon in lieu of an alcoholic beverage. In refusing dessert you can say, "No, thank you, but I'd love some of that great coffee you make." In this way you don't leave the person making the offer with his foot in his mouth. Offering an alternative helps to smooth the interaction.

CHANGING THE SUBJECT

On some occasions, particularly when someone is being persistent, try to change the subject. Start discussing business, fishing, current events, the weather, or anything. Anything but cigarettes, food, or alcohol, that is. If you're at a social gathering, bring other people into the conversation. If someone is especially persistent, continue to refuse and then leave his presence. However, it is unlikely that anyone, except perhaps an intoxicated host trying to get you to have one more for the road, will be too pushy once you say "No" the first or second time. Of course the easiest method at a cocktail party is to have a drink in your hand. No one will know what's in the drink, so that if you decide to have plain seltzer no one will be the wiser. Also, no one will bug you about having a drink.

EYE CONTACT

One of the most basic yet most essential elements of a refusal response is direct eye contact. When you refuse while looking someone in the eyes you convey the message that you really mean what you're saying. If refusing an offer of this nature makes you feel ill at ease, you might have a tendency to avoid direct eye contact. You might look at the ceiling or floor or to one side. You must practice looking directly at people when refusing. You can begin by looking at people more frequently in everyday conversations. Remember, you can also overdo it. *Don't stare.* People who are very socially skilled and assertive have developed this skill well. In fact, direct eye contact can be used to intimidate others by putting them on the defensive. Even in the animal kingdom the dominant animal will stare down his opponent until his adversary gives up.

Women are frequently more adept than men at eye contact. Several years ago my colleagues and I conducted studies on married couples. Husbands and their wives were instructed to talk to one another for twenty minutes while we recorded their interactions on videotape. Ratings of the nonverbal interactions revealed that wives consistently looked directly at their husbands more than the husbands looked at their wives. In fact, each husband very seldom looked directly into his spouse's eyes when talking to her. In the area of nonverbal assertiveness women are far superior to men.

EMOTIONAL EXPRESSION

Unless you give the impression that you are really serious about what you're saying, no one will pay much attention to you. Your expressiveness is conveyed through (1) the tone of your voice, (2) your facial expression, and (3) body language and gestures. Your voice should be firm, with a tone loud enough to indicate you mean what you say. Do not pause, stammer, or hesitate. Do not break the flow of your remarks with "uhs" or "ahs." I'll illustrate this point with a couple of examples. Read the following statement hesitantly, and in a low tone of voice.

> "Well, ah . . . Margaret . . . ah . . . I know you went to a lot of trouble to prepare this . . . but . . . ah . . . I . . . ah . . . really shouldn't."

Now read the following remark in a firm voice without pausing.

> "Margaret, I know you went to a lot of trouble to prepare this but I *definitely must* refuse."

There's quite a bit of difference, isn't there? You're saying almost the same words each time, but the way you say them makes all the difference in the world.

Now, what about your facial expression? A common mistake people make is to smile when they are saying "No." Smiling is a cop-out! For example, if you smile when you complain to your spouse about something he or she is doing to annoy you, you're really conveying the message, "I'm only half serious about what I'm saying, so don't get mad or upset." You water down your responses when you smile and lessen their impact. On the other hand, you don't have to frown or look angry either. After all, you're simply refusing an offer of a cigarette, drink, or food.

PRACTICE MAKES PERFECT

In teaching people new behavior patterns in clinical practice, a variety of techniques are used. Training includes a step-by-step process in which an individual

1. Learns the components of the new behavior pattern
2. Observes a role model engaging in the behavior pattern
3. Rehearses the response under simulated conditions
4. Views his reactions on videotape
5. Receives feedback from others on the adequacy of his performance
6. Rehearses the response repeatedly until performance is adequate
7. Practices the new response style in real-life situations

Now, pretend that a particular situation is actually happening. Imagine that your aunt or your friends are there facing you and have made you an unacceptable offer. Refuse their offer. Be firm. Refuse in a strong, serious tone of voice. Don't smile. Use your body, arms, and hands to get your message across. Look straight ahead. After you're finished, rate your performance on a scale from 1 to 10, keeping in mind the following guidelines:

Rating	*Performance*
9–10	Excellent: voice quality and body language used well
6–8	Generally good, but needs some practice on eye contact, voice quality, affect, or body language
3–5	Below average: forgot to include all of the verbal elements of the planned refusal response; nonverbal elements poor

| 1–2 | Poor: response was too brief and choppy— noticeably nervous, speaking rapidly; affect, body language, and eye contact poor |

If you rated yourself anything less than 9 or 10, determine what elements are most in need of improvement. Then work on each element, one at a time. If you were learning to play golf, you'd probably concentrate on one component of your swing at a time. You'd become confused if, as a novice, you tried to think about keeping your head down, elbow in, and other rules during each swing. You might end up not doing any one of these things and completely missing the ball. The same is true of refusal skills. For example, if eye contact is one of your problems, practice your refusal response concentrating *only* on looking straight into the mirror. Remember, practice only one element at a time until you have mastered it. Then move on to the next, and the next, until your over-all performance is worthy of a 9 or 10 rating.

It will be helpful if on at least a few occasions you can enlist the aid of a partner to practice with you. He or she can play the part of the host or aunt and give you the opportunity to practice under slightly more realistic conditions. Besides, you are not only practicing the mechanics of *what* to say and *how* to say it but you're emotionally conditioning yourself to feel more at ease when you refuse. To do this you must instruct your partner to be as persistent and persuasive as possible, to use every trick in the book to get you to give in. Then, if you can handle that, you can handle anything.

SECOND AND THIRD RESPONSES

While in most cases your initial refusal will be effective, some people may counter your refusal with a second request that you overindulge. Don't be dismayed. Simply reply with a second refusal similar to the first. You must be a bit more firm in your tone of voice with the second refusal. A third or fourth offer by someone will necessitate a minor confrontation. You'll need to say something such as:

"Your persistence won't change my mind. Please stop offering me a drink, Milt. *I positively don't want one.* Your constant insistence is irritating."

At that point, turn and become involved with someone else. If you are at lunch or otherwise unable to get away, quickly change the topic of conversation.

PLANNING AHEAD OF TIME

It is helpful to avoid offers of food, alcohol, or cigarettes by letting people know ahead of time that you will be abstaining or consuming very little. For example, you can very easily inform your hostess, when you are invited to a dinner party, that you will not be able to eat certain foods. Most people will understand, especially if they are prepared in advance. At a business lunch you can avoid remarks encouraging you to have a drink by setting a nondrinking standard. Be the first to order, and ask for a cup of coffee before lunch instead of a cocktail. By sounding eager for the coffee you'll keep others from encouraging you to drink. For example, "I'm just dying for a good hot cup of coffee" or "I'm so thirsty—I'd like a large glass of ice water before lunch."

Beware—The Modeling Effect

In addition to tempting you through direct social pressure, other people have a more subtle influence on your behavior through a phenomenon known as *modeling*. Modeling refers to a social imitation process whereby you tend to behave in a manner similar to that of people around you. The influence of other people's behavior on yours will vary depending on who they are and how you perceive them. We are more likely to model the behavior of people who are similar to us in appearance, mannerisms, age, and background. We are also more likely to model people whom we hold in high esteem or who are friends of ours. This is a far-reaching process that occurs without our awareness. I'm sure that if you gave it some thought you would find that you have picked up certain mannerisms from your spouse or close friends without realizing that *modeling* was responsible. Modeling can even influence your preferences and attitudes. It has been found, for example, that high school students taking an interest inventory expressed more preferences for military careers when the test administrator was a military man dressed in uniform than when a civilian administered the test.

The smoking, drinking, and eating of those around you can have a definite effect on your own habit pattern. Smokers, for example, are much more likely to smoke while interacting with other smokers. Studies have also indicated that when you smoke in the presence of other smokers you are likely to smoke more than you would if you were with nonsmokers. You would even be prone to take more puffs and inhale more deeply.

Modeling of eating patterns is a little more complex and is much more dependent on the individual. While some people are influenced to eat more in the presence of an overeater, others actually eat much less under such conditions. You may find that when people are overeating, you give yourself more excuses to eat, or, as the transactional analysts would say, you give yourself permission to eat. On the other hand, you may be a solitary eater. You may eat next to nothing when with others, perhaps out of embarrassment. Many people who are overweight feel extremely self-conscious about their eating habits. They often believe that others are watching them eat and perhaps saying, "Look at that fat woman. You'd think she'd know better than to eat so much food." If you are this type of individual, you may be relatively impervious to the eating style of others. Overeating by others may, in fact, have the reverse effect on you—that is, you might eat less.

Several behavioral studies have demonstrated a strong modeling effect when alcoholic beverages are being consumed. In one study by Dr. Alan Marlatt and his colleagues, heavy social drinkers were asked to participate in a taste-rating task during which they would drink wine and rate its taste. They were told to drink as little or as much as they wanted. Certain subjects were given this taste test in pairs. Unknown to the real subject, the other subject in each pair was one of the experimenters. With some subjects the experimenter drank a great deal of wine (a full bottle) while making his ratings; with other subjects he drank very little (3 to 4 ounces). A number of subjects were given the taste test alone. The object of the study was to determine if being in the presence of a heavy drinker influences an individual's drinking rate. The results of the study were dramatic. Subjects exposed to the heavy-drinking model drank over twice as much as subjects exposed to the light-drinking model. The latter group actually drank much less, about 25 percent less, than subjects who took the test alone.

It is clear that the drinking habits of those you associate

with have a powerful influence on your behavior. You may even have noticed this phenomenon when you're at cocktail parties, small social gatherings, or business lunches. You must be aware of this influence and consciously fight it. As you drink, notice if you are drinking at a faster or slower pace than those around you. Make sure you pay attention to both your drinking *and* their drinking. In fact, to insure your own moderate drinking, you should begin to associate more with light and moderate drinkers and avoid very heavy drinkers. Give some thought to your closest friends and business associates. Which ones are heavy drinkers? Has their drinking ever influenced yours? Make a definite commitment to recognize modeling influences and to choose your drinking associates accordingly.

Another way of coping with modeling effects is to make a challenge out of being the model for others. Try to influence others, through your actions, to drink less or at a slower rate. You can do this without their being aware of your intentions. The next time you're drinking with someone else, begin to pace your drinking rate to match your companion's. When he or she takes a sip, you take a sip. If the other drinker takes a large sip, you take a large sip. Now, after a few minutes, start to slow down your drinking rate. Pace your drinking so that you're taking about half the number of sips that your companion takes. Let twice as much time go by between your sips and his. Also, make certain you take much smaller sips than he does. Now, observe his behavior carefully. Is his drinking rate changing? Is he slowing down? In order to be successful with this modeling procedure, your companion must be closely involved in conversation with you. He must be paying attention to you. Thus, in addition to realizing the effects of modeling on your drinking, you can begin to influence the influencers. Who knows? You may change all your friends into controlled, moderate drinkers without saying a word to them.

Other "Friendly Enemy" Maneuvers

In addition to direct social pressure, other people may affect your habit-control efforts in more subtle ways. Pessimistic comments from others will start your own negative thoughts working. If enough people tell you that success is impossible, you'll begin to believe them. Maybe not at first. But their attitudes will rub off on you and very subtly influence your thoughts and actions. You'll think, "Maybe she's right. Maybe I should give up this whole program and resign myself to the fact that I'll never be able to change." If you happened to be somewhat discouraged before the comment was made, the remark will only serve to reinforce your discouragement. That is, sometimes you'll be able to handle these comments better than at other times. However, you should be prepared to handle them *all* the time.

Also, comments that do not support your efforts will upset you, depress you, and generally hurt your feelings. You'll feel sorry for yourself. One of your greatest enemies is feeling sorry for yourself. When you have tried to control your habits in the past, have you ever said, "What's the use? Nobody appreciates what I'm doing anyway. People give me a hard time whether I'm trying or not."

You must be specific in telling (teaching) a person exactly what he or she says and does that makes it more difficult for you to control your habit. Here are examples of *good* teaching versus *poor* teaching.

Example 1: Poor Teaching
"Gloria, you make me mad, and that drives me to smoke. I wish you'd cut it out."

Example 2: Good Teaching
"Gloria, when you criticize me about my smoking, even though I'm really trying to quit I get frustrated and annoyed. I realize that I'm more likely to smoke when I have these feelings. It would help me an awful lot if you wouldn't criticize my efforts."

The statement in Example 1 serves to antagonize rather than to teach. The remark is argumentative; it blames Gloria not only for making you mad but for making you smoke. The tone is harsh and abrupt, and it is highly unlikely that Gloria will cooperate. She's likely to get defensive and say something else to make *you* angry again. Also, the statement provides little information about what Gloria does to influence your smoking. The phrase "you make me mad" doesn't indicate anything about Gloria's behavior. She must be told specifically *what* she does to make you mad.

In Example 2 the spirit of the comment is positive. You are very matter-of-factly telling Gloria what she says that angers you. Instead of blaming her for your smoking, and thereby putting her on the defensive, you're merely pointing out the relationship between your anger and your smoking. Finally, you ask her in a reasonable way to change her behavior.

You can provide even more clarification by giving one or two specific examples of instances in which she was critical. You could say

"Gloria, remember last Saturday night, when we were out with the Hudsons? Well, I was lighting a cigarette, and it was only my second one that day. You said, 'Can't you show some self-control just for one day?' I thought your comment was unfair and I got angry. Remember? I went and bought another pack of cigarettes and smoked the rest of the evening."

Just state the facts as they occurred. Don't add any side remarks, such as "See! You really don't want me to quit smoking, do you?" Such statements are childish and unnecessary. They are also extremely unproductive. Remember that your goal is to lessen someone's negative influence on you. You want that person to change his or her behavior. Keep thinking of yourself as a teacher and you'll be okay.

One of the most essential elements of your teaching is to instruct your student *what* to do differently. It is not enough to point out the things he or she says that trigger your habit. You must teach your student what to do instead. For example: "George, instead of teasing me about my diet, why not let me know you appreciate my efforts? A kind word or a hug every once in a while when I'm doing well would really mean a lot to me." To be effective you *must*

1. Be specific.
2. Stay calm.
3. Provide examples.

Let's discuss several examples of friendly enemies and how to handle them, using the principles I've just described.

Case Examples

ELLIOT

Elliot and Crawford have been good friends and neighbors for seven years. They live next door to each other in Hasbrouck Heights, New Jersey, and commute to New York each day by train. Elliot is a forty-year-old president of a large electronics firm. He is a self-made man, who rules his company

210 PERSONAL HABIT CONTROL

with an iron hand. His word is law, and he does not tolerate anyone's questioning his judgment. At home he has a difficult time relaxing. He worries constantly about his business even though the company's profits are increasing substantially each year. His tendency to rule his family as he does his business has caused much turmoil. His wife appeases him but is depressed most of the time. His children try to avoid him and are looking forward to the day when they'll be going off to college.

Crawford is so much different from Elliot that people often wonder how they can be such close friends. Although they are the same age, Crawford looks about five years younger than Elliot. Crawford is vice-president in charge of production for a large clothing manufacturer. He has an easygoing manner, and his success has been built on his friendly, sincere way of relating to other people. Crawford, his wife, and teenage son have a very close relationship. He considers himself a family man first and a businessman second.

Crawford and Elliot play golf together every Sunday, and about once a month they and their wives play bridge or eat dinner together. Since they are next-door neighbors they frequently have passing conversations as they're coming or going.

Everything between the friends was going smoothly until Crawford decided to quit smoking. He felt that it would be better for him to reduce smoking gradually, so using the Personal Habit Control program, he set up a very systematic plan for himself. He set a target date for complete abstinence of February 15, one month away. His program included (1) gradually eliminating cigarette consumption in specific locations (for example, while driving a car, while watching television), (2) using a muscle-relaxing routine and calisthenic exercises to reduce urges to smoke, and (3) practicing various thought-control motivational techniques (described in Chapter 6) every day.

At golf Crawford happened to mention to Elliot that he was trying to give up smoking. Elliot was quite interested, so Crawford told him in great detail about his habit-control strategy. As Crawford progressed with his description he could tell by the look on Elliot's face that his interest was turning into dismay. The conversation then went as follows:

Elliot: "Crawford, let me give you a little advice. I don't mean to tell you what to do, but . . . you're going about this the wrong way."

Crawford: "I don't understand."

Elliot: "Well, first of all, your system will never work. Nobody can quit smoking gradually. You've got to go cold turkey. That's the way I did it ten years ago, and that's the *only* way to do it."

Crawford: "But, you don't understand, I read that some people find it easier to quit gradually and are more successful that way. This psychologist said—"

Elliot: "That's a lot of bull. What the hell does a psychologist know anyway. The guy probably never smoked in his life. Now, look, I'm serious—if you don't give them up completely, right now, you might as well forget it."

Crawford: "But I'm really learning what situations control my smoking and what triggers my urge to smoke."

Elliot: "That sounds like a lot of nonsense to me. It's simply a matter of willpower. Take me, for example. I have total control over myself at all times. You just don't have as much willpower as I do. You've got to be a man about it, Crawford."

> *Crawford:* [*annoyed*] "Elliot, this has nothing to do with being a man. I—"
>
> *Elliot:* "Look, I've never known anybody who was able to quit smoking doing it your way. You're just kidding yourself. Just wait. In a few days you'll be telling me that I was right and you were wrong."

After their conversation they each went home. Crawford felt frustrated and annoyed. Elliot *always* had to be right. He could usually handle Elliot's overbearing manner, but today he felt intimidated by him. He thought that what Elliot said made sense in a way. Maybe he *was* going about it the wrong way. After all, Elliot had quit smoking and had never started up again. He should know what he was talking about.

With this mixture of frustration, anger, and self-doubt, Crawford lit a cigarette. After that he lit another one. As he smoked he thought, "Boy, look at this. Smoking two cigarettes in a row. Elliot must be right. I *don't* have any willpower. Oh, hell! I can't quit smoking. I'll be damned if I'm going to continue to torture myself like this." Crawford was very much affected by Elliot's remarks. Rather than see the connection between smoking and Elliot's comments, Crawford fell into the trap of blaming himself and his supposed lack of willpower. The real influential sequence of events, the antecedents of smoking, went as follows:

Elliot's negative remarks ⟶ annoyance ⟶ anger ⟶ self-doubt ⟶ negative expectancies about success ⟶ smoking

Now let's run that scene over again, except that this time Crawford will handle Elliot's negative comments more appropriately.

Crawford: "Elliot, I'm more enthusiastic about this
method than anything else I've ever tried. It
makes a lot more sense."

Elliot: "Crawford, let me give you a little advice. I
don't mean to tell you what to do, but . . .
you're going about this the wrong way."

Crawford: "I'm sure this is the *only* way for me to do it."

Elliot: "Well, first of all, your system will never
work. Nobody can quit smoking gradually.
You've got to go cold turkey. That's the way
I did it ten years ago, and that's the *only*
way to do it."

Crawford: "Elliot, everyone has to find his own way to
quit. The cold-turkey method worked for you,
but this is better for me. A lot of people quit
gradually. Besides, by quitting gradually I'm
learning what situations control my smoking
and what triggers my urges to smoke."

Elliot: "That sounds like a lot of nonsense to me.
It's simply a matter of willpower. Take me,
for example. I have total control over myself
at all times. You just don't have as much willpower as I do. You've got to be a man about
it, Crawford."

Crawford: "Elliot, I know you mean well by your advice, but your remarks aren't helping me. I
know my way will work *for me.* I *know* that
willpower, as you describe it, has very little to
to do with it. Look, Elliot, your *advice*
is making it harder for me to keep a positive
attitude. I've found out that I need
encouragement, not advice. Let's make a
deal that *you* won't advise me again on how
to quit smoking. I need your help as a
friend—so how about it?"

Elliot: "I'm merely trying to give you the benefit of
my experience."

Crawford:	"I realize that, Elliot, but I've tried a lot of ways to quit smoking. While I'm quitting with this method I *must* believe in it totally and have no doubts. So, in the future, no advice and no negative comments. When you say, 'You just don't have as much willpower as I do,' it discourages me. I begin to doubt myself."
Elliot:	"Okay, pal, whatever you say. But if you ever need my advice, just ask. I can't say I still won't have my doubts, but I'll keep them to myself."
Crawford:	"Thanks for trying to help."

In this dialogue Crawford maintained a firm, positive attitude throughout. He did not let himself be put on the defensive. He rationally challenged Elliot's arguments without getting upset. He gave direct instructions to Elliot on how he wanted him to help. He didn't instruct him in a hostile or defensive way but asked him as a friend to be more encouraging. Notice that Crawford did *not* try to convert Elliot to approving of his method of habit control. This is not necessary, and such attempts often lead to unending and useless argument. In fact, at the end of the conversation Elliot said that he'd still feel the same way but simply wouldn't say anything. This is sufficient. All Crawford needs is that Elliot refrain from offering advice on smoking. Encouraging remarks would be helpful, but *no* remarks would do. You must learn to compromise when asking other people to change their behavior to suit your needs.

GINGER

Ginger and Nancy are thirty-six-year-old identical twins living in Philadelphia. They grew up in Dayton, Ohio, the daughters of a Methodist minister who was a strict disciplinarian. Their mother was a rather quiet, passive woman, but very affectionate. Both girls were overweight as children and have battled the bulge throughout their lives. Ginger is five feet six inches tall and weighs 175 pounds, while Nancy is slightly shorter and weighs 186 pounds.

Ginger is divorced and lives alone. She manages a florist's shop and enjoys her work. Ginger is a rather reserved and moralistic individual who is very conscious about the "proper" way to live one's life. She leads a quiet existence and has few friends. Her greatest joy is the frequent meetings with her sister for lunch or dinner. Food is a major element in her life and she prides herself on being a gourmet cook. She constantly *thinks* about food, *dreams* about food, and *talks* about food.

Her sister Nancy is unmarried and teaches the fourth grade at a local elementary school. She is a shy, reserved person, a studious type who likes to read a lot. Lately she has felt very lonely and dissatisfied with her life. Because of her weight she stays by herself most of the time and has no close friends. Her main social interaction is with her sister when they frequently get together for a meal.

After a great deal of thought Nancy decided to stop feeling sorry for herself and do something about her life. She decided that she must lose weight once and for all. Rather than go on another fad diet (she'd tried diets to no avail), she set out to change her eating habits permanently, using Personal Habit Control. She considered *what* she eats, *how* she eats, and all of the possible things that trigger her desire to eat. After a month of dieting she had lost 25 pounds and was feeling great. She really felt in control of herself. She wanted to get down to 130 pounds. As she lost weight she began to take more of an interest in her appearance and in other people. She began bicycling and walking. She even invited two other teachers to the movies one evening.

As her diet progressed, Nancy realized that her relationship with Ginger was changing. In fact, Ginger's constant discussion about tempting foods made things more difficult for her. The more weight Nancy lost, the more critical Ginger became. She frequently made comments such as, "Nancy, you don't need to lose any more weight" or "You're not as much fun anymore" or "Nancy, these clothes you're wearing since you lost weight are just not right for you." Nancy discovered that she often overate after such comments.

In addition, Nancy found it more and more difficult to avoid overeating when she was with Ginger. It seemed as though nearly every time they got together, food was a major focus. Ginger *always* served snacks or dessert when Nancy visited her and she was constantly wanting to try out a new gourmet dish or a new specialty restaurant. She *insisted* that Nancy join her in eating high-calorie foods.

Nancy decided that unless she changed the nature of this relationship she would not succeed in achieving permanent control over her weight. As the first step she told Ginger that her constant discussions about food and insistence that she eat too much were very frustrating to her. She pointed out that she could control her eating in just about every situation *except* when she was with her. Nancy tried to stress the importance of her commitment to change her eating habits and over-all life style, and she pointed out the negative influence her sister was having on her. Specifically, she asked Ginger (1) *never* to offer her food under any circumstances and (2) *never* to discuss appetizing foods, new restaurants, recipes, or food matters in general with her. To Nancy's amazement, Ginger readily agreed. She honestly hadn't thought Ginger would understand since she was usually extremely defensive about personal criticism.

Nancy's amazement didn't last long, however, because less than one week later Ginger was doing exactly what Nancy had asked her not to do. In fact, she seemed to be talking about food even more and bringing more pressure to bear on Nancy to join her in overindulging.

In the past Nancy would probably have given up at this point, figuring there was nothing she could do about her sister. She might have continued to have this problem and perhaps forgotten about her diet because of it. But this time was different. She was determined that she would not let anything or anybody stand in her way. She felt that if she didn't change her appearance and her life *now,* she'd never do it. In evaluating Ginger's influence on her, Nancy realized that she was most likely to overeat when she and Ginger were at Ginger's house or when they ate a meal together. To help her conceptualize the details of a solution to this antecedent problem she wrote out the following plan of action:

1. At least temporarily, I will not visit Ginger at her house or eat meals with her.
2. To do this I must be firm in refusing invitations from Ginger.
3. As a substitute I will (1) invite Ginger to my house and serve only noncaloric beverages or low-calorie food and (2) invite Ginger to non-food-oriented activities, such as going for a walk or a bicycle ride and attending the theater or a performance of the symphony orchestra.

On the following day Ginger called Nancy and asked her to go to a new restaurant with her. Nancy politely refused and suggested instead that they meet later to go bowling. Ginger became very insistent about the restaurant. Nancy then told Ginger very straightforwardly that she could *not* continue to eat with her anymore because it threw her off her diet. She added that she wanted to continue their get-togethers, but the circumstances of their meetings would have to change. Ginger felt hurt and upset and responded with "If that's the way you feel, let's forget the whole thing. I don't know what's come over you lately. You're being hateful and I haven't done anything to you. You should never have started this diet. It's not good for you. You're not the same person anymore."

Nancy was upset for the rest of the evening. She didn't want to hurt Ginger. She hadn't meant to hurt her, but Ginger's reaction made her feel guilty as hell. "Maybe Ginger is right," she thought. "Maybe I'm not the same person anymore since I'm on this diet." Then it dawned on her that she *wasn't* the same as she used to be and that was *good*. That's what she wanted. She wanted to lose weight *forever*, and in order to do it, she had to change herself. Actually, Ginger had given her encouragement without realizing it.

The next day was Saturday, so she went over to Ginger's apartment to straighten things out. The conversation went like this:

> *Nancy:* "Ginger, I want us to be able to get along with each other. But I must have your cooperation in changing my habits."
>
> *Ginger:* "I think all this dieting is silly. You'll gain it all back anyway. What difference does it make if I have you over to dinner once in a while?"
>
> *Nancy:* "It makes a big difference. In the past all we used to do was eat and talk about food. I can't do that anymore. I want more out of life than food."

Ginger: "You'll ruin your life, Nancy. After you lose all that weight you'll be going out more, staying out late. You'll probably even have men pestering you all the time."

Nancy: "But that's just what I want! I've been sitting around letting my life pass me by. I'm bored, bored, bored with my life. I'm lonely. *Fat* and lonely. And if you were honest about it, you'd say the same thing about yourself."

Ginger: "What? Me? I'm perfectly happy with my life."

Nancy: "Oh, come on, now. I think the fact that I'm losing weight and going out more with friends is upsetting you. I think that in a way you're jealous of my success. Be honest with me, Ginger."

Ginger: [*crying*] "I hate to admit it, Nancy, but you're right. At first I didn't think you'd lose weight. I thought you'd last about two weeks on the diet and then gain it all back. Then I saw you were succeeding, and it scared me. I was afraid we'd gradually lose touch with each other. And, yes, you're right, I am jealous. Seeing you lose weight and keep it off made me realize that it *could* be done. I had convinced myself that you and I were just naturally fat and there was nothing that could be done."

Nancy: "Well, why don't we lose weight together?"

Ginger: "No, I'm not ready for that yet. But I *will* try to help you. Just tell me what I can do."

Nancy again detailed what was needed, and they both agreed to it. Although Nancy felt sorry for her sister, for her unreadiness to change, she felt personally confident in her own abilities to change her habit patterns once and for all.

STANLEY

Stanley and Ruth live on Long Island and have been happily married for thirty-three years. Ruth, fifty-six, is a rather short (five feet three), heavyset woman who has had a weight problem for about fifteen years. As a young woman she was described by her friends as "petite" and was often complimented on her slender figure. Her weight problem bothered her a few years ago, but now she's resigned to the fact that she is overweight and probably always will be. As a wife, mother, and grandmother she enjoys preparing good food and eating it as well. Since her eldest son and his family live close by, she has on hand a steady supply of cookies, cakes, fudge, and brownies for her two grandchildren. She nibbles constantly, testing her culinary delights.

Stanley has been concerned about Ruth's weight for several years. He has difficulty in understanding her plight since he's as skinny as a rail and can eat anything he wants. He is convinced that Ruth has no willpower and that the only way she'll lose weight is for her to be strictly supervised. He realizes that she resents anybody telling her what to do, but he feels he knows what's best for her. After all, she's been on every diet imaginable but has never stuck to any of them for more than a few days.

In addition to her weight problem, Ruth hasn't been feeling well lately. She's been having dizzy spells and periodic pains in her chest, and finally went to the doctor. Dr. Eisler, their internist, asked to speak with Ruth and Stanley together after he had completed Ruth's physical examination. He told them that Ruth had very high blood pressure, and with her weight and family history of heart problems, she was a prime target for a stroke or heart attack. He impressed upon them the absolute necessity of Ruth's losing weight and keeping the weight off. He spoke sharply and purposely frightened both of them.

After Dr. Eisler's conference with them Ruth was determined to lose weight. Although he didn't mention it, Stanley was just as determined to take charge of Ruth's weight-reduction program. Soon after Ruth began the dieting Stanley began examining her plate at each meal and calculating the exact number of calories. He kept a running account of his figures in a notebook. At the end of each day he lectured Ruth on what "mistakes" she was making on the diet. "The way I figured it," he would say, "you were a hundred calories over your limit today." At first this amused Ruth. At least, she was amused until Stanley began to intensify his supervision. He brought home diet books for her to read. He cut articles on dieting out of the newspaper or magazines to give to her. He began planning their menus and accompanying her to the supermarket to make sure she bought only what was on the list. He would not allow her to bake any more of her cakes and pies.

Ruth found herself getting more and more irritated with Stanley's "help." She had begun the diet with a great deal of enthusiasm, but now she felt as if she were being treated like a two-year-old. She resented Stanley's interference and began eating out of spite. She ate secretly when he was out. She'd sneak cookies into the house and hide them away until an opportune moment when Stanley wasn't around. Her motivation to lose weight was completely shattered. The more she ate the stronger her appetite became. Of course she was concerned about her health, but the threat of a heart attack seemed so remote. "It won't happen to me," she thought.

An incident at a local restaurant convinced Ruth that she couldn't go on in this way. She and Stanley were out with close friends, celebrating Stanley's birthday. Ruth was giving her order to the waitress, trying to be careful about calories, when Stanley loudly interrupted her. "No, no, Ruth, that's all wrong. Miss, I better order for my wife. She'll just have a salad with no dressing and broiled fish with no butter," he said. Stanley then turned to their friends and said, "Ruth has absolutely no willpower. I have to treat her like a child when it comes to food." Everyone had a good laugh *except* Ruth. She was so embarrassed and hurt she didn't know whether to burst into tears or throw something at Stanley.

That evening after Stanley went to bed she had a long talk with herself. She knew she *had* to lose weight. She also knew that Stanley was making it impossible for her to lose. He was driving her crazy! She decided to settle the matter once and for all.

Early the next morning at breakfast Ruth pointed out to Stanley what he was doing to her.

Ruth:	"Stan, I've got to talk to you about my diet."
Stanley:	"Good. I've been meaning to talk to you about the way you were ordering at the restaurant last night. I—"
Ruth:	"Now, wait a minute, Stan! That's just what the problem is. I am *not* a baby. I do *not* need you to order for me. Look, honey, I know you're trying to help me, but your constant supervision of my diet is backfiring. I resent it. In fact, I sneak foods just to spite you."
Stanley:	"You *what?*"
Ruth:	"Now, let me finish! You are *embarrassing* me and making me feel like a child. I realize that I haven't had any control over my eating in the past. But this time, if you'll help me, I can do it. Maybe I should say 'if you *don't* help me.' Stan, you're just too much involved."
Stanley:	"Ruth, I'm just trying to help."
Ruth:	"I know that. But you're *not* helping. The more you supervise me, the more I eat. It's not working."
Stanley:	"Well, what do you want me to do?"

Ruth: "I *must* be in charge of my own diet. I do think it would help me to weigh in at the doctor's office once a week. I need to report to *some-body*. I think that'll help me. I would rather that you weren't involved, Stan. Just encourage me and praise me when I'm doing well, but ignore anything else. Even if I happen to eat a little bit too much of something. When you mention it, I just eat more. Let's take last night, for example. Your remarks were uncalled-for. Will you promise to help me?"

Stanley: "Okay, we can try it your way. I guess I didn't realize what I was doing to you."

Ruth: "Now, Stan, let's make sure we understand each other. Let's lay down same ground rules. First, no counting my calories. Second, no more articles or books on dieting. Third, *I'll* plan my meals, *not you.* Fourth, no ordering for me when we're out. Fifth, no comments about my diet to anyone else. If I want to discuss my diet, *I'll* bring it up, not you. Of course an encouraging remark from you once in a while would be really helpful. Make *positive* comments, not negative ones. Tell me how well I'm doing or how much thinner my face looks. Is it a deal?"

Stanley: "Sure, it's a deal. I was just worried about you. I'll do whatever you say as long as it helps you lose weight."

In each of the above cases the successful approach to the "friendly enemy" was a direct one. Specific feedback was provided on what needed to be changed. Avoidance of the issue will only make matters worse.

Take Your Own Advice

You must remember that just as it is difficult for you to change your smoking, drinking, or eating habits, it's equally difficult for your "friendly enemies" to change their behavior. After all, they've probably been reacting to you in the same way for years. *Don't* expect them to change overnight. They may comply with your instructions *most* of the time but have a slipup every once in a while. In the case of Ruth and Stanley, for example, he may "forget" and perhaps say, "Ruth, are you sure you're allowed those kind of vegetables on your diet?" Ruth can respond in one of three ways. She can ignore his comment, in which case he may fall back into his supervisory role again. She can raise hell with him for not keeping his promise. This is likely to cause friction and turmoil and generally be unproductive. Finally, she can simply point out that he is falling back into his old pattern and ask him to try harder. She can respond with "Oops! You're becoming my supervisor again, Stan." No admonitions are necessary. Stan will get the point and will probably appreciate her not making a fuss. After all, she's asking *him* not to make a fuss over her diet.

The most important aspect of taking your own advice is to maintain a positive approach to others. Be aware of episodes in which your "friendly enemies" are really trying to change their responses. When they encourage you or refrain from questioning you, point it out. You might say, for example, "I really appreciated your not saying anything to me tonight when I ate a baked potato. I know it's difficult to change, and you're helping me out a lot."

Remember, take a positive attitude toward others and reward them when they change their behavior. The more frequently you openly recognize appropriate support from others, the more frequently you'll receive it.

CHAPTER NINE

─── Getting Started

You are now ready to put my Personal Habit Control system to work for you. Since the beginning of your program will be the most difficult time for you, I'll provide a step-by-step guide to get you through the first few days.

When Should You Begin

Since giving up a habit can be very traumatic, you might have a tendency to avoid starting your habit-control program. Don't make excuses. *Begin immediately*. If you put it off until next week, you're likely to put it off again when next week rolls around. *Your starting date should be the first morning after you finish reading this book*. Keep the book handy and use it as a reference, especially during the first two to three weeks.

Which Habit Should You Break First

Let's suppose that you eat, drink, *and* smoke too much. Where should you begin? Should you try to control these habits all at once or work on them one at a time? I suggest that you choose only one habit to work on at a time. Giving up two or three habits together is simply too stressful for most people. Start with the habit that will be the easiest to break. Decide which is your least addictive habit. Rate the strength of your cravings for food, cigarettes, and alcohol separately on a ten-point scale. The higher the score, the higher your average craving. Now examine which habit is the strongest in terms of how much and how frequently you consume. Choose to break the habit that has the *lowest* craving score and the *lowest* quantity/frequency level. Do not attempt to modify your second or third habit until the first one is under control. This will take at least six to eight weeks.

Of course you may choose to begin controlling a particular habit over the others because of an immediate health risk. If your physician has advised you to quit smoking because of an acute medical condition, then by all means start with that habit.

Some habits are difficult to separate from one another, since changing one necessitates changes in another. A good example is the influence of weight control on alcohol consumption. You *must* reduce alcohol consumption while dieting simply because alcohol contains unnecessary calories. You also must drink less while dieting, because alchohol interferes with inhibitions and self-control and frequently triggers eating episodes. After two drinks at a cocktail party you may say, "To hell with my diet. I'm going to have a good time tonight and eat whatever I want."

Keep in mind that changes in one habit can also have a negative influence on other habits. The most common example is the effect of quitting smoking on weight. Since many people experience a 15- to 20-pound weight gain when they quit smoking, you must be prepared for this eventuality. The best method of dealing with this problem is to prevent its occurrence. You do *not* have to gain weight when you quit smoking. It is not inevitable. You will gain weight only if you use eating as a substitute for smoking. In addition, since food tastes so much better when your taste buds are not clogged with smoke, you're likely to eat more after you give up cigarettes. If you use activity and exercise as substitutes for smoking and make certain that your eating pattern stays the same, you won't gain weight. In fact, a major advantage of my Personal Habit Control system is that it is applicable to all habits. Therefore, when you quit smoking with the aid of my thought-control techniques or Personal Relaxation Training, you can readily apply these same techniques to your eating behavior. In fact, most people who have used my system notice that when changing one habit they actually gain *more* control over other habits.

How to Prepare Yourself

Before your starting date, prepare yourself by purchasing index cards, graph paper, a pedometer (to measure physical activity), and, if you'll be dieting, a good scale. Most bathroom scales are not very accurate since they are influenced by changes in humidity and temperature. I use an electronic, digital readout scale that weighs to the tenth of a pound and is extremely accurate. I suggest that you buy either one of the electronic scales designed for home use (the Counselor 77 model is available from J S & A National Sales Group, Department TL, One J S & A Plaza, Northbrook, Illinois, 60062) or a good, heavy-duty bathroom scale.

Remember, your *starting* day will *not* be the day you reduce or eliminate your habit. You *must* spend the first week monitoring your behavior as I have discussed in Chapter 3.

Use your index cards to record consumption patterns, and transfer the information to a graph. Resist the temptation to skip this self-monitoring phase. It is extremely important and will be of tremendous help to you. Monitor your behavior for one week, seven full days. *Do not begin to reduce or eliminate your habit until this self-monitoring is completed.*

You can also prepare yourself during this week by giving some thought to alternative activities that can serve as substitutes for your habit. In Chapter 4, I discussed the importance of changing your routine, particularly at times of the day when you're most likely to overconsume. Prepare a list of possible activities, hobbies, and exercises that you'll be using. If any of these activities requires equipment, buy it this week. For example, you may need to buy a sketch pad, paints, a jump rope, an exercise bicycle, modeling clay, crossword puzzles, woodworking tools, or knitting supplies. Don't put this off. Have your list and your materials ready and available for next week.

The Day Before You Begin

On the final day of your self-monitoring week examine your records carefully. Determine what specific situations, times of day, thoughts, feelings, and people trigger your habit. Reread Chapter 3 and set specific behavioral goals for yourself. Start out slowly. Establish goals only for the first 24 hours. Specifically, the day before you begin to quit or reduce your consumption you should

1. Set habit-control goals just as Dorothy did in Chapter 3. Include consumption goals, such as "I will limit myself to 1,000 calories, divided into three meals, with no snacks," *and* Personal Habit Con-

trol goals, such as "I will practice Personal Relaxation Training twice a day."

2. Plan your schedule for tomorrow, hour by hour. Write this schedule out and keep it handy. Change your normal routine as much as possible. Spend as much time as possible in low-probability antecedent situations (Chapter 3). Do not leave any unstructured time. Follow your schedule faithfully!

3. Discuss your habit-control plan with family and close friends. Give them specific instructions on how they can help. Reread Chapter 8 to refresh your memory.

4. Remove all unnecessary temptations from your surroundings. Give snack foods away or place them in inaccessible locations in your house. Destroy or give away all cigarettes or alcohol if you will be abstaining completely. Remove all ashtrays from your view. Keep cigarette and liquor supplies to a minimum if you are decreasing your consumption.

5. If you are gradually decreasing cigarette or alcohol consumption, with abstinence as your future goal, set your *quitting* date. Your quitting day should be no longer than three weeks away. Write the date on a card and place it in full view of everyone at home and/or at the office.

6. If you will be controlling your weight, plan menus for all meals for tomorrow and make certain that all necessary low-calorie foods are available.

The First 24 Hours

The first day that you actually quit or cut down on your habit is a critical one. You must be prepared with a definite plan of action. I have outlined below a specific step-by-step plan for the first 24 hours of your habit-control program for smoking, overeating, and drinking, separately. Follow this plan faithfully.

THE FIRST 24 HOURS
SMOKING

Morning
1. Wake up 20 minutes early.
2. Practice Ultimate Consequences Technique (Chapter 6) for 10 minutes.
3. Breakfast: substitute tea or juice for coffee.
4. Keep index-card record all day of strong urges and/or cigarettes smoked; include time, situation, feeling, and Personal Habit Control technique used to control behavior.
5. Follow schedule set previous day; avoid high-probability smoking situations.
6. Remove ashtrays and cigarettes from surroundings.
7. Practice Personal Relaxation Training (Chapter 5) for 15 minutes in midmorning.
8. Limit coffee drinking to one cup in the morning in "safe" situations (with nonsmokers or where cigarettes are not available).

Afternoon
1. Lunch: avoid alcoholic beverages.
2. Follow schedule set previous day.
3. Practice Covert Conditioning (Chapter 6) in mid-afternoon and whenever cigarettes are in view.

4. Use deep breathing, fist clenching, and relaxation (Chapter 6) to control urges to smoke.

Evening
1. Avoid alcoholic beverages before dinner.
2. Dinner: limit yourself to one glass of wine, if any.
3. Take vigorous walk, bicycle ride, or calisthenics for 30 minutes to one hour in midevening.
4. Review records and assess progress; review any negative thought patterns during the day (Chapter 6).
5. Record on graph urges and number of cigarettes smoked.
6. Set goals for tomorrow based on progress today (reread Chapter 3).
7. Plan to reward yourself tomorrow morning for reaching your goal today—e.g., buy something special, call a friend and brag, schedule a tennis match, read a chapter in a favorite book. (Do *not* use food as a reward!)
8. Reread Chapter 4 on self-control.

In Addition, if You Are Quitting Gradually
1. Eliminate smoking in two situations (e.g., while driving, while in the kitchen).
2. Practice *controlled* consumption (Chapter 7) by taking shorter puffs, longer time between puffs, and fewer puffs.
3. Smoke only three-quarters of each cigarette.
4. At least on three occasions put your cigarette out after two puffs.
5. Keep only half a pack of cigarettes available to you

at any time; give the rest to your spouse or a friend or keep them in an inaccessible location.

THE FIRST 24 HOURS
WEIGHT CONTROL

Morning
1. Wake up 30 minutes early.
2. Weigh yourself and take measurements (chest, waist, hips); write information on weight graph. (Weigh and take measurements only once per week.)
3. Dress and practice Ultimate Consequences Technique (Chapter 6) for 10 minutes.
4. Set pedometer to zero and attach to belt or pin at waist.
5. Breakfast: practice new eating style (Chapter 7) —self-monitor *before* eating; take smaller bites, put fork down between bites, eat slowly.
6. Keep index-card record all day of food eaten, calories, time, situation, feeling.
7. Follow schedule of morning activities.
8. Practice Personal Relaxation Training (Chapter 5) for 15 minutes in midmorning.

Afternoon
1. Lunch: practice your new eating style.
2. Follow schedule of afternoon activities.
3. Walk for 30 to 40 minutes in midafternoon.
4. Use Covert Conditioning (Chapter 6) and relaxation to control urges.
5. Review negative thought patterns during the after-

noon; write negative thoughts ("This will never work") on index card and write positive alternatives next to them.

Evening
1. Practice exercise routine or walk 30 minutes before dinner.
2. Take no alcoholic beverages before or during dinner.
3. Dinner: practice new eating style. Discuss habit-change progress with family.
4. Avoid usual routine; avoid kitchen.
5. Engage in two new alternative activities, interests, or hobbies after dinner.
6. Practice Personal Relaxation Training 20 minutes before retiring.
7. Review records and assess progress; review negative thought patterns (Chapter 6).
8. Set goals for tomorrow based on progress today (reread Chapter 3).
9. Record pedometer miles and write on activity graph.
10. Plan to reward yourself tomorrow morning for reaching your goal today—e.g., buy something special, call a friend and brag, schedule a tennis match, read a chapter in a favorite book.
11. Reread one chapter in this book; choose a chapter pertaining to an area giving you difficulty.
12. Praise spouse, family, or friends for "appropriate" support during the day; discuss interactions still in need of change.

THE FIRST 24 HOURS
DRINKING

Morning

1. Wake up 30 minutes early.
2. Practice Personal Relaxation Training (Chapter 5) for 20 minutes.
3. Have breakfast.
4. Keep index-card record all day of strong urges and/or alcoholic beverages consumed; include time, type and amount of beverage, situation, feeling, and Personal Habit Control Technique used to control behavior.
5. Follow schedule set previous day.

Afternoon

1. Lunch: eat with someone who knows you are breaking your drinking habit or eat in a restaurant that does not serve alcoholic beverages.
2. Follow afternoon schedule.
3. Practice Ultimate Consequences Technique (Chapter 6) for 15 minutes in midafternoon.
4. Use Covert Conditioning (Chapter 6) and relaxation to control urges.
5. Avoid all contact with alcohol stimuli (e.g., bars, liquor advertisements, conversations about drinking, liquor stores).

Evening

1. Avoid all parties and social gatherings where alcohol is served.
2. Walk, bicycle, or exercise (calisthenics) during the hours before dinner.

3. Eat dinner at least 30 to 60 minutes earlier than usual.
4. Practice nondrinking alternative activities (e.g., go to a movie, read, draw, write letters—keep busy).
5. Avoid rooms of the house and sitting areas where excessive drinking has occurred.
6. Reread one chapter in this book; choose a chapter pertaining to an area giving you difficulty.
7. Review records and assess progress; review negative thought patterns (Chapter 6).
8. Record on graph number of urges or number of ounces of alcohol consumed.
9. Set goals for tomorrow based on progress today (Chapter 3)—e.g., what Personal Habit Control techniques you should use. Reread Chapter 3 if necessary.
10. Plan to reward yourself tomorrow morning for achieving your goal today—e.g., buy something special, call a friend and brag, schedule a tennis match, read a chapter in a favorite book.
11. Discuss progress and/or habit-control problems with spouse or close friend; praise family for "appropriate" support.
12. Practice Personal Relaxation Training before retiring to induce sleep.

In Addition, if You Are Quitting Gradually
1. Set a limit on the number and types of drinks allowed (Chapter 4); should not be more than 5 ounces of liquor, 12 ounces of wine, or 3 cans of beer in any 24-hour period of time.

2. Practice *controlled* consumption (Chapter 7) by
   taking smaller sips, mixing weaker drinks, taking
   more time between sips.
3. Never finish a drink—always leave at least one
   ounce.
4. Concentrate on internal sensations associated with
   different amounts of alcohol consumption (Chapter 7).

The First Few Weeks

Once you've gotten through the first day, you'll feel a lot
better. There is something about the first 24 hours that is
extremely stressful for most people. After all, giving up your
habit is like giving up an old friend.

During the first week continue to plan your routine and
follow a definite schedule, just as I have outlined for the first
day. Practice the Personal Habit Control techniques daily.
Plan a definite time each day to practice specific techniques.
Develop as many alternative activities as possible to serve as
substitutes for your habit. Don't let up, especially during the
first week or two. After the first two weeks your schedule can
be more flexible. However, continue to use your new habit-
control skills at every opportunity. After a few weeks most of
these skills will become so habitual that you'll be doing them
automatically.

Unless you are abstaining completely from your addiction,
continue self-monitoring your behavior for at least one month.
Then monitor your consumption only periodically, a few days
each month, to assess your progress. If you are abstaining,
you need to monitor urges for only a week or two or until
their frequency and intensity subside.

As the days and weeks pass by, you'll feel less tense and more in control of your habit. You'll have survived the ordeal. Because you've developed new self-control habits in the process, you'll feel very self-assured and confident. *You,* and not a cigarette, alcohol, or food, are now in control of your life.

CHAPTER TEN

<u>Permanent</u> Personal Habit Control

When you first begin a new habit-change program you are extremely enthusiastic. You're totally involved and highly motivated. It's a little like being a recent convert to a religion or political ideology. Your own enthusiasm, the support of your family and friends, and the novelty of the Personal Habit Control system itself keep your motivation strong.

Just be careful. A point may arrive when the appeal of the method begins to wear off. Your family will begin to take your efforts for granted, and your enthusiasm will wane. This is a critical period of time, which may occur anywhere from one to six months after you begin your program. Don't be alarmed when this happens. It's perfectly natural. However, the way in which you react to this drop in motivation may well determine the permanence of your habit change.

How many times have you gone on a diet and simply become bored with it? Habit control can become a drudgery, a dull routine, *if* you let it. Do not focus all of your attention on the number of pounds you've lost, number of days or weeks since your last cigarette, or number of drinks you've had this week. Certainly these things are important, since they represent your ultimate behavioral goal. But too much daily emphasis on overconsumption or lack of it will cause you to feel deprived. You'll feel miserable, as if you're missing out on something that everyone else is enjoying. Don't emphasize your deprivations, but rather focus on your newly acquired self-control skills. Emphasize the new ways of thinking and behaving that you are learning. Concentrate on *positive* alternatives to your old habit. This positive, comprehensive approach provides you with a continuing challenge that will sustain motivation over a long period of time.

While the right attitude is essential, you still will have trouble with Personal Habit Control from time to time. You'll find yourself periodically slipping back into your old habit. Perhaps you won't actually smoke, eat, or drink in excess, but you'll give it a lot of thought. If you expect trouble and plan for it, you'll overcome it.

Let's examine several techniques that will remotivate you. When your commitment to habit control wavers, consider the following:

1. Reevaluate your habit by keeping written records of urges and/or consumption.
2. Try all the habit-control techniques I have recommended.
3. Plan regularly scheduled self-assessments of your progress.
4. Arrange for a buddy to help you.

Do not

1. Blame yourself.
2. Tell yourself you're a failure.
3. Blame your trouble on lack of willpower.
4. Blame somebody else.
5. Give up.

Self-Assessment

Whenever the going gets rough, the first thing to do is to take a giant step *backward*. Go back to the beginning to determine exactly what the trouble is.

Refer to the discussion of self-observation in Chapter 3 and again keep an accurate, daily record of your consumption. Write down *what* you are consuming, *when, under what circumstances,* and *with whom.* If you've given up alcohol or cigarettes completely but find yourself weakening, make a record of your urges. Under what circumstances are they occurring? At what time of the day? What thoughts or emotions are triggering cravings? What people are influencing you?

Examine these records and refer to them often. During the course of self-monitoring you'll discover that you will automatically recover your momentum. You might merely have been getting a little lax with your habit-control efforts and needed some constructive feedback. Behavioral feedback is an important element of habit change, yet because it's so simple many people underestimate its value. Continue periodic self-assessment at least once a month. It will not only get you out of your slump but also pinpoint trouble spots.

One of my overweight patients who must lose 80 pounds has kept on her weight-control program using just this procedure. Whenever her willpower begins to fade (which happens about once every three to four weeks), she immediately starts a daily eating diary. Since she usually becomes less active when she starts to eat more, she also wears a pedometer every day and keeps an exercise and activity diary. She then hangs up large graphs of her daily caloric intake and pedometer mileage in a conspicuous place in her kitchen. Almost immediately she's out of her slump and off and running, both figuratively and literally. After three or four days this feedback is no longer necessary. Her eating diary, graphs, and pedometer are always handy just in case she should need them.

The Habit-Control Inventory

Sometimes feedback via self-assessment is insufficient to re-motivate you. Perhaps you're not using all the Personal Habit Control techniques available. Perhaps you're not using them often enough or at the appropriate times.

You must evaluate the habit-control techniques you're using and how you're using them on a regular basis. Permanent habit control can only be achieved by consistent effort. To insure consistency during the first week of your program you should assess your efforts at the end of each day. For the next three months evaluate yourself once per week. After that, assess your progress at the end of each month for a year. That's right! You must continue to evaluate your efforts on a monthly basis for one full year.

To assist you in this evaluation process I have devised the "Habit-Control Inventory," which you should complete at each evaluation time. The inventory is printed below.

Habit-Control Inventory
Which of the following habit-control techniques have you used in the past week? *Give specific examples of how you used them.*

1. *Thought-Control Techniques*
   _____Yes _____No

2. *Changing Antecedents of Consumption*

_____Yes _____No

3. *Changing Consequences of Consumption
   (Rewards)*

_____Yes _____No

4. *Personal Relaxation Training*

_____Yes _____No

5. *Exercise and Recreational Activities*

_____Yes _____No

6. *Changing Consumption Style*

_____Yes _____No

7. *Support from Others*

_____Yes _____No

244 PERSONAL HABIT CONTROL

Notice that the inventory includes the major areas of emphasis of the Personal Habit Control system. Make certain you are honest with yourself when responding to each category. Also, *be specific*. Do not check "Yes" to any category unless you can list specific instances in which you used that procedure. For example, under the category *Changing Antecedents of Consumption* a dieter might check "Yes" and then list the following:

1. I only eat at the kitchen table.
2. High-calorie foods and snack foods are kept out of the house.
3. From 5:00 to 6:30 P.M., when I used to eat snacks and have a couple of drinks, I write letters, read, or refinish furniture.

Under *Thought-Control Techniques* a smoker might list:

1. I have used the Ultimate Consequences technique several times this week to control urges to smoke.
2. At the end of each day this week I have made a list of any negative thoughts or rationalizations I've used that might sabotage my progress.

By examining your self-monitoring records along with the inventory you can easily see where you need improvement. For example, you may discover that during the past week you have been overeating whenever you are tense and rushed. In looking over your responses to the inventory you may find that you checked "No" to the categories *Personal Relaxation Training* and *Changing Consumption Style,* two maneuvers designed to deal specifically with the problem you're facing. Get busy and set goals for the next week in each of these areas. You can write these goals on the Habit-Control Inventory sheet under the appropriate categories. In this way you can evaluate your successful application of these techniques at your next evaluation session. In each of these categories your goals might include the following:

> *Personal Relaxation Training*
> 1. I will practice relaxation training for 20 minutes each day next week.
> 2. I will use a brief muscular and deep-breathing relaxation exercise before each meal.
>
> *Changing Consumption Style*
> 1. At every meal I will practice eating more slowly, taking smaller bites, and putting my fork down between bites.
> 2. To remind myself to slow down I will place a timer on the table and set it for 20 minutes for each meal.
> 3. I will ask my husband to slow his eating style to help me remember to slow mine.

In addition, look over your inventory responses to each category. What techniques are missing? What additional procedures could you be using? If you check "No" to any one category during two consecutive evaluation sessions, reread the chapters in this book pertaining to those techniques. Perhaps there are some habit-control strategies that have slipped your mind, and reading a chapter or two will refresh your memory.

Also, ask yourself what excuses you're using for not putting certain techniques into practice. Too busy? Someone else's fault? Too many temptations? Be honest, now. You know none of these are good excuses. In fact, I have provided you with specific ways of dealing with these situations throughout the book.

The Buddy System

If you're having trouble, perhaps "going it alone" is your problem. You may be the type of individual who functions best with group support and mild social pressure. You may be able to control your habit better if you can report your progress to somebody. If so, you can arrange a buddy system, with either one other person or a group. Be sure you choose a good friend, someone who is understanding. Don't choose a relative, especially one you live with. The best person to choose is someone who is also controlling a habit or who has successfully learned to control a habit in the past. Set up a system in which one of you calls the other every few days. During the first week or two of your program you may want to call daily, say at 10:00 P.M every evening. During the conversation report your progress. Describe the habit-control techniques you've used and exactly how and when you used them. The thought of having to make that call and "confess" to overconsumption will be a great deterrent. However, these conversations should not be censorious in nature. If you slip up, discuss ways in which you could have controlled your habit. Use your mistakes as learning experiences. Your buddy should keep a positive attitude, giving advice and offering suggestions. Simply having someone to talk to who understands what you're going through will help.

You should also arrange an emergency-call system, so that you're able to call your buddy when you need quick advice or when you're being tempted. Alcoholics Anonymous uses this technique very effectively.

You may want to form your own group of habit controllers. Group support and encouragement can be an invaluable aid. Such groups as TOPS (Take Off Pounds Sensibly), Alcoholics Anonymous, and Overeaters Anonymous are built on this principle. While I am a strong advocate of peer support, I must warn you that it's only an adjunct to your other efforts. You must use the basic habit-change procedures I've described and use them consistently in order to succeed. Group support merely helps to reinforce you and insure that you apply these procedures consistently.

A number of years ago Dr. Leonard Levitz and Dr. Albert Stunkard, of the University of Pennsylvania, conducted a study of TOPS, the self-help group for dieters. TOPS is not a commercial venture such as Weight Watchers but is a non-profit self-help program. Weekly sessions conducted by the group members themselves include a weigh-in, an announcement of weight gains and losses, group support and encouragement, and a general discussion of dieting. Over 200 members from sixteen different TOPS chapters were involved in this study. Drs. Levitz and Stunkard wanted to determine if group support alone could be an effective weight-control procedure or if specific habit-control techniques are also needed. During the study TOPS members received one of four different treatments: (1) self-control techniques taught by a professional, (2) self-control techniques taught by a TOPS leader, (3) nutritional education conducted by a TOPS leader, and (4) the usual TOPS program. The self-control techniques were similar to some of those described in Chapter 4. The results indicated that self-control techniques were *essential* for weight loss. A one-year follow-up showed that, on the average, those who had received only group support (with or without the nutritional education) gained their weight back. Dieters in the group receiving self-control techniques taught by a profes-sional were the most successful. Thus while group support can encourage you, don't rely on it as your sole method of habit control. Use it as one of the many techniques in your armory.

Continued Problems

Let's suppose that even after you implement the techniques I've described you continue to have problems in controlling your habit patterns. Unfortunately, in some cases *self*-help can go only so far. You may need more intensive help, perhaps even professional help.

Studies examining the immediate and long-term results of habit-control programs have helped to pinpoint factors responsible for success or repeated failure. For example, Dr. Ovide Pomerleau and his colleagues at the Center for Behavioral Medicine at the University of Pennsylvania recently completed a detailed analysis of 100 cigarette smokers. All of these smokers participated in an 8-week smoking-control program. At the conclusion of the 8-week course, participants who were completely abstinent from cigarettes were compared with those who were still smoking. As compared to the successful ones, those who failed were those who, at the beginning of the program,

1. Had smoked for a greater number of years
2. Had smoked more cigarettes per day
3. Were more overweight
4. Failed to consistently use the self-control techniques they were learning in the program

The first two factors indicate that smoking control is more difficult if your habit is extreme or chronic. The same is true of eating behavior. People who have been overweight since childhood are the least likely to succeed at dieting. This doesn't mean that you're a hopeless case if you've been over-weight for a very long time. It simply indicates that your habit is complex and you've had more years to practice it. You must be even *more* vigilant and *more* consistent in your efforts than other people.

Heavy drinking follows the same pattern. Persistent consumption of large quantities of alcohol over a period of years will make habit control difficult. Such drinking affects your total life and health, which complicates the change process. In addition, physical addiction to alcohol may necessitate professional and medical assistance. While many experts differentiate between social drinking, problem drinking, and alcoholism on the basis of certain "symptoms," you really don't need to categorize yourself. Basically, these labels represent the degree of severity of your problem, which in turn helps to predict the chances of your success. Just remember that the more severe your drinking problem in terms of (1) the amount you consume, (2) the number of years of heavy consumption, and (3) the effects of drinking on your life, the more likely you are to need professional help. In fact, a generally accepted definition for alcoholism is alcohol consumption that significantly interferes with interpersonal, occupational, marital, emotional, or physical functioning in your day-to-day life. You don't have to be concerned with diagnosing your own problem. All you need to consider is that if you are unable to reduce or eliminate your drinking using self-help techniques, you need a professional to help you achieve your goal.

In addition to the severity of your habit, certain characteristics about *you* may be important in determining ultimate success. In Dr. Pomerleau's study, failures at smoking control did *not* consistently apply the techniques they learned. In fact, many of them did not keep daily records of their cigarette consumption for even one day. You *must* implement these techniques for them to work. There is nothing magical about learning a self-control procedure. You must work at habit control. In the beginning you must work hard. If you put in the effort at the beginning, habit control becomes easier as time goes on. Your *new* healthy habits become so much a part of you that you won't even have to think about them.

Depending on the severity of your habit-control difficulties, you may need the professional help of a physician, psychologist, or psychiatrist. I would suggest you choose a professional who is experienced in the behavioral sciences, who has an orientation of behavior therapy or behavior modification. These are often psychologists, many of whom are members of the Association for the Advancement of Behavior Therapy (420 Lexington Avenue, New York, New York 10017). Behavioral psychologists in private practice, hospitals, clinics, and colleges and universities treat habit-control problems using both individual and group approaches.

Checklist Review

To review what you've learned about Personal Habit Control, test yourself on the questions below.

1. Before starting your habit-control program have you observed and monitored your habit pattern for at least a week?

   _____ Yes _____ No

2. Have you reviewed your self-observation records looking for High- and Low-Probability Antecedent Clusters?

   _____ Yes _____ No

3. Have you set specific behavioral goals that you can realistically achieve?

      _____Yes   _____No

4. Are you emphasizing changes in your habit *patterns* rather than in the amount of substance you're consuming?

      _____Yes   _____No

5. Have you rearranged your surroundings to decrease temptations?

      _____Yes   _____No

6. Have you planned enjoyable alternative activities for times of the day when you're most likely to overindulge?

      _____Yes   _____No

7. Are you rewarding yourself for positive habit changes?

      _____Yes   _____No

8. Have you tried using a behavioral contract?

      _____Yes   _____No

9. Are you practicing Personal Relaxation Training on a regular basis?

      _____Yes   _____No

10. Are you using Personal Relaxation and thought control to overcome episodes of emotional overconsumption?

      _____Yes   _____No

11. Have you established a regular schedule of exercise and recreational activities?

      _____Yes   _____No

12. Do you refuse offers of food, cigarettes, or alcohol assertively?

_____Yes _____No

13. Have you practiced the elements of an appropriate refusal response so you feel comfortable with it?

_____Yes _____No

14. Have you instructed your "friendly enemies" how they can help you?

_____Yes _____No

15. Are you continuing to provide positive feedback to your "friendly enemies" when they try to help you?

_____Yes _____No

16. Have you changed your consumption response style?

_____Yes _____No

17. Are you practicing the "ultimate consequences" technique regularly?

_____Yes _____No

18. Are you continually reviewing excuses you make to deviate from your Personal Habit Control plan?

_____Yes _____No

19. Have you practiced positive statements to counteract your excuses?

_____Yes _____No

20. Are you regularly reviewing your progress with the aid of the Habit-Control Inventory?

_____Yes _____No

If you've answered yes to the majority of these questions, you're doing well. If not, you'd better get going. Remember, you must put *all* of my techniques into practice to be successful.

Ultimate Success

If you stick to it and really develop these Personal Habit Control techniques, you *will* succeed. Your self-management skills will become your new habits, your *healthy habits*. You'll also experience a side benefit of this method. You'll begin to feel personally powerful over not only your habits but your life in general. The skills you've learned will be useful in other aspects of your day-to-day existence. The ability to relax, control your thoughts, deal more effectively with other people will be continued assets. Just remember: practice these new healthy habits and they'll be with you forever. And forever, in terms of your life span, will be a lot longer because of successful habit control.